Health
in Early
Childhood
Settings

From Emergencies
to the Common Cold

'One must ask children and birds how cherries and strawberries taste.'
Johann Wolfgang Goethe

For Frania. And for Brandon and Brooke.

Let us give the world to the children at least for one day
Let them play with it as if it is a spangled balloon
Let them sing and dance among the stars

Let us give the world to the children
Like a huge apple or a warm loaf of bread
at least for one day
so that they'll have enough to eat

Let us give the world to the children
so that even if it's for one day
it will learn what friendship is

The children will take the world
out of our hands
and they will plant immortal trees

Nazim Hikmet
Translated by Prof Talat S. Halman

Health in Early Childhood Settings

From Emergencies to the Common Cold

Professor Frank Oberklaid

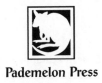

Pademelon Press

First published in 2004 by
Pademelon Press
7/3 Packard Avenue
Castle Hill, New South Wales, 2154

Editing and Project Management by Persimmon Press
Design by Tania Edwards
Typeset by Sun Photoset, Brisbane
Index by Forsyth Publishing Services
Printed in Australia by Ligare Pty Limited

© Frank Oberklaid

Oberklaid, Frank.
    Health in early childhood settings: from emergencies to
    the common cold.

    Includes index.
    ISBN 1 876138 17 3.

    1. Child care services - Health aspects. 2. Day care
    centers - Health aspects. 3. Children - Health and hygiene.

    362.712

Foreword

Early childhood, the early years, has emerged as a major focus of attention for governments and for researchers across a range of disciplines. This interest has seen a growing commitment from governments towards policy initiatives that foster the healthy development of young children.

Alongside this interest in the importance of the early years has been an increase in the number of children who are experiencing non-parental care arrangements from a very early age. These arrangements include settings such as centre-based day care, family day care and preschools. In terms of outcomes for children's developmental health and wellbeing, it is essential that these environments provide young children with high quality experiences.

One of the biggest challenges to providing good quality early childhood environments is ensuring the health and wellbeing of children. While there has been ongoing debates concerning the key elements of quality, a consistent finding from extensive research has been the importance of health factors as a key indicator of quality and predictor of positive outcomes for children.

Drawing on his extensive knowledge and experience, Professor Frank Oberklaid, one of Australia's leading paediatricians and early childhood advocates, has written an invaluable authoritative resource for early childhood practitioners and for parents.

Health in Early Childhood Settings — From Emergencies to the Common Cold is a very accessible, easy-to-follow publication dealing with the common health issues busy practitioners face on a daily basis in their work with young children and their families.

The author adopts a broad view of health to include developmental, behavioural and social emotional aspects. Early childhood services need to address the preventative as well as the psychosocial aspects of health as important components in the provision of high quality care.

The book emphasises the context in which children develop. This includes the child in the context of the early childhood setting, the family, and the child and family within the context of the community in which they live. The early childhood practitioner is encouraged to develop strong links with all elements that make up the child's contextual environment, with particular emphasis on working in partnership with families and health care professionals in the local community.

Health in Early Childhood Settings — From Emergencies to the Common Cold is a welcome addition to the early childhood literature. I commend the book to all who are concerned about providing healthy environments for our young children. While the book is primarily for people working with young children in a range of environments, it is also an excellent resource for early childhood students, policy makers and for parents.

June Wangmann
Director, NSW Centre for Parenting and Research, Department of Community Services

Contents

Introduction

This book is written for those people whose work involves them with infants, toddlers and young children; this includes early childhood settings such as child care, family day care, kindergartens and preschool, and the early years of school. Parents may also find this book useful as a brief but accurate guide to the common health, developmental and behavioural problems of young children.

This is not designed to be a comprehensive account of all the illnesses and problems faced by young children; there are other books that have been written for that purpose. Rather, it provides information about the more common issues and problems of childhood.

It has been written with the busy practitioner in mind. The layout of the book is intended to make it easy to locate individual topics, and it is written in what I hope is an open, user-friendly style.

For most topics, the content is organised into easy-to-follow and intuitive headings: cause, signs and symptoms, treatment or management, when to seek medical advice, and prevention (when appropriate and relevant). The topics are organised into body systems to make them easy to find, though not all topics fit neatly in this way. For example 'obesity' is in the section on gastrointestinal, whereas it could easily be in a section of its own.

An attempt has been made to provide some sort of perspective on the prevalence and importance of certain conditions. For example, the section on asthma is many times longer and more detailed than the section on pneumonia. Asthma is very common in young children and it is probable that every early childhood setting will have children with asthma, whereas pneumonia is relatively uncommon and the child is likely to be in hospital or at home rather than in a community setting. Conditions like polio, diphtheria and tetanus are not mentioned at all because they are not seen in our community at all these days due to the success of immunisation.

People will use the book in different ways. Some will read topics or sections of interest; others will look up a topic or check the index when the need arises, for example when they are looking after a child who is sick or who displays some symptoms or signs. In this situation one can use either the Table of Contents or Index to quickly locate a topic or keyword.

I have made a conscious decision not to be specific about a number of issues. For example, I have not specified when parents should be notified; this is usually a matter of commonsense and will vary according to a number of factors, such as the age of the child, the perceived severity of the symptoms, how confident the staff are in managing common problems, the wishes of the parents, and access to good and immediate advice from a nurse or doctor. As indicated above, many of the topics have sections on treatment and when to seek medical advice. This is not to imply that the readers of this book should either take responsibility for treatment, nor for seeking medical advice. Rather, the topic is organised in this way so that the reader will come to understand the condition itself and be more informed about health aspects of young children.

This book is designed to be a useful and practical resource for all those places where young children congregate. However, there are some things this book is not intended to be:

▶ It is not comprehensive in the sense of listing all childhood illnesses or symptoms.

▶ It does not attempt to provide all the details of the clinical features, treatment or management of a particular condition or problem. It provides enough information for the professional or parent to develop an understanding of aspects of the condition, the cause, the principles of treatment, and when to seek medical advice.

▶ Books of this kind, no matter how credible and comprehensive, should *never* be used as a substitute for specific medical advice. The information here can help guide and inform but, at the end of the day, if you have any concerns at all about the health of the child you should always share this with the parents and suggest they seek appropriate medical advice. A good relationship with knowledgeable and caring health professionals is very important for parents and for those entrusted with the responsibility of caring for or teaching young children.

Gender balance

at the English language does not have a gender neutral 'she'. In my previous book, I used 'he' exclusively, as being neutral and apologising to those who took book, I have interspersed 'he' and 'she' throughout the This is also not very satisfactory, but I trust that you will for it as you read.

▶

children we are referring to developmental, behavioural and more traditional view of health. Recent years have seen a of illness and injury and other health problems. There e early identification of problems and their early ork with young children, even those without a health t role to play in prevention and early detection. In ip they have with parents, they are in a unique verbalise and ventilate their concerns regarding their em the child's uniqueness and strengths. They can formation as well as other forms of support, and als when appropriate.

A word about settings

In every community there are a range of professionals who work with children. One of the problems with the way the service system for young children is organised and funded is that there are few incentives for coordination and communication, so that mostly services tend to operate in isolation from each other. *I encourage those working in early childhood settings with children to make contact with the health professionals in their community.* Some communities have regular meetings of professionals working with young children — child and family day care workers, preschool teachers, community and maternal and child health nurses, general practitioners, and so on. It is no surprise to find that where this happens, professionals are more confident in being able to address health, developmental and behavioural issues in children. They feel they are working as part of a team, and can obtain support and advice when it is needed. Further, they are aware of resources in the community where they can refer children and parents for further assessment as needed.

Early childhood professionals are often the first to notice a problem, or else the first person the parent turns to if they have a concern. This may be to do with simple issues such as viral infections or school sores, or more serious problems such as asthma or some other chronic illness. Often they are to do with concerns about development, such as delayed speech or difficulty following instructions. They may have to do with concerns such as poor socialisation or aggressive behaviour. In such cases it is good to know who in the community deals with these sorts of problems, especially when they are beyond what can be reasonably managed by the early childhood professionals. Clearly, the child's general practitioner is often the first port of referral, but for some issues the maternal and child or community health nurse may be appropriate, as might other professionals. Some child care centres and kindergartens undertake a 'mapping' exercise so they know all of the agencies and individuals in their community who can provide support in terms of advice or referral.

It is a good idea to do this anyhow. Find out information about general practitioners, community nurses, pharmacies, paediatricians, hospitals, family support and other relevant agencies in the immediate community. Here is a checklist of people, agencies and phone numbers that might be useful. Type this up and keep it near the telephone or in a place where it is prominent and everyone knows where to find it:

▶ poisons information centre;
▶ ambulance;
▶ police;
▶ fire brigade;
▶ hospital;
▶ children's hospital;
▶ general practitioner;
▶ maternal and child health/community nurse;

‣ pharmacist;
‣ local government health department; and
‣ others.

The importance of an identified general practitioner

All children benefit from regular contact with a general practitioner for management of the invariable minor and occasional more serious illnesses of childhood. The doctor comes to know the child and the family, and parents come to trust the advice given. A mutual, trusting and informed partnership between parents and health professionals provides the best chance of optimal health outcomes.

Foundations of Health

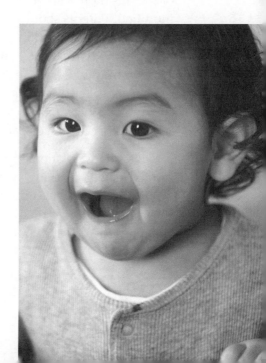

Building a relationship with the child's parents

As one of their key goals, all professionals who work with children should have the development of a good relationship with the child's parents. Leaving young children in the care of another person is always a difficult thing for parents to do. It involves a degree of trust and an acknowledgment of the professional's training and competence. Implicit in this trust is an expectation that the child will be cared for or taught in a competent, sympathetic and sensitive manner.

Once this trust is established, the professional is sometimes expected to extend themselves beyond their normal duties and be a friend, counsellor, confidant, the person to whom the parent can turn to for advice about any aspect of the child's health development or behaviour, a source of knowledge about resources for the child and family, and more. Sometimes parental expectations can be impossible to meet. Professionals working with children need to be very clear about their roles and their level of skills and expertise in relation to the child or to family issues that may come up. Sometimes it is important to explicitly state the boundaries of the parent–professional relationship.

Nevertheless, early childhood professionals working in early childhood settings can play an important and often very significant role in the life of the young child. They do have a perspective and a level of expertise that the parent may not have. They have the benefit of often many years of experience with young children. They spend a lot of time with the individual child, and have the opportunity of observing her across a diverse range of daily situations; they have a unique opportunity to observe the child as a uniquely developing person, her interests, passions, competencies and relationships. Because of this, they are often the first to be concerned that a child may not be communicating well, or may have a hearing problem, or delayed language, or difficulty relating to other children.

Parents may seek advice about a child's development or behaviour, or may be able to observe as the professional models the way in which a child's language can be stimulated or socialisation with other children encouraged, or difficult and challenging behaviour modified. Parents should be encouraged to raise any concerns with the professional, and in turn those working with young children should establish the kind of trusting relationship that allows a mutual sharing of observations and any concerns. The Centre for Community Child Health in Melbourne has produced a resource to facilitate this kind of sharing called *Sharing a Picture of Your Child's Development.* This can be ordered from the Centre by calling (03) 9345 6150, or by sending an email to the following address <enquiries.ccch@rch.org.au>.

This sort of relationship is likely to lead to positive outcomes for the child and the family, as well as being very satisfying for the professional. It can be promoted by formal structured regular meetings in which the child's progress is discussed, or by simple informal exchanges on a day-to-day basis. Simply sharing a little titbit about the child's day with the parent when the child is picked up is always of interest to the parent, as is keeping a piece of work the child has done. All parents are keen to hear how their child is progressing, but also want to learn about how their child spent the day — what she did, whom she played with, whether she ate her lunch, and so on.

Creating a health profile for each child

It is useful to create a 'health profile' for every child. This can be done at the time of enrolment and updated each year or when circumstances change. Ask the parents to complete a simple questionnaire about the health of their child. This should include information about any previous health conditions that may be relevant; any current health problems or things they are concerned about; any condition that requires ongoing treatment; medications that the child needs to take on a daily basis; anything else the early childhood setting needs to know, such as allergies, special diets, or anything else that may necessitate special treatment or precautions. Included in this profile should be exact details of who to call if the child gets sick, or in an emergency.

For children who have a chronic medical condition, this information is especially important. If the child has asthma, then a written 'asthma action plan' should be available; this lists the regular medications that the child takes, and gives exact instructions as to what steps to take, including specific medications and doses, if the child has an acute attack of asthma.

Sometimes a letter from the child's doctor is helpful, both in terms of explaining the nature of the condition, the treatment, and any special instructions to the staff. It is very important that everyone understand in considerable detail the condition itself and the implications for the particular setting, whether it is child care, family day care, preschool or school. It is also extremely important to share information on the child's understanding of his condition, the gestures and terminology he uses to describe symptoms, the way he best copes with the condition, and the way parents ask him about symptoms. It is worthwhile sitting down with the parents so that this information is shared and both parties are clear about management in this setting.

Medications

A surprising number of young children are on medications of one type or another. Sometimes this is a short-term course, lasting a matter of days, and sometimes longer. A small number of children with a chronic medical condition need to take medications every day. Make sure that everybody is very clear about use of medications. There are regulations and accreditation guidelines for storage and administration of medications. These include keeping medications in a safe place that is inaccessible to young children, preferably a locked cupboard; storing them in their original containers clearly labelled with the name of the child; giving them at specified times, and so on.

There is increasing concern over the unnecessary use of medications in young children, both those obtained by prescription and those that can be bought over the counter from a pharmacy. Many children who have simple viral infections are inappropriately prescribed antibiotics. These do not work in such situations and may have unpleasant side effects. In recent years there has been a national education campaign directed at doctors in an attempt to decrease the prescribing of antibiotics and other unnecessary medications.

However, doctors worry also about the high number of children who are given over-the-counter medicines. These include simple analgesics and anti-cold medications, medicines to help the child sleep, vitamins and natural remedies given for a host of reasons. Most of these medicines are unnecessary. While it is not suggested that early childhood professionals enter into detailed discussions with parents about the pros and cons of a particular medication for an individual child, they can and should query the need for giving them, and ask that a letter be obtained from the child's doctor.

Medicines are discussed further throughout the book in sections covering specific conditions.

Alternative therapies (complementary medicine)

Recent years have seen a literal explosion of interest in alternative or complementary therapies. Surveys show that instead of consulting doctors, nurses, pharmacists, or allied health professionals, more and more people are seeking advice from practitioners who practise complementary medicine. Many people choose a combination of Western medicine and complementary therapies, and the number seems to be growing rapidly. The situation is the same for children. After years of mostly dismissing these therapies as ineffective and potentially dangerous, many universities and medical schools now have research programs into complementary medicine. It is now commonly held that at least some of them show promise of being of benefit in the treatment of a range of conditions.

There is a group of health care providers in the community who come from a variety of backgrounds. Some undergo comprehensive training programs, which can be as long as three or four years; others simply set up shop with very little in the way of training. Few barriers exist in the way of persons who want to provide services to those with health problems, as long as they do not represent themselves falsely; for example, by claiming to be a doctor or nurse. Generally they are free to treat consumers (including children) in any way that is acceptable to themselves and to their patients. They provide a large variety of therapeutic modalities, ranging from massage to special diets, and from vitamin supplements to colonic enemas.

The most pressing research questions are to find out, amongst the numerous and diverse range of therapies, those which are effective or promising and those which are of no benefit or even harmful. For children this is an even more pressing need, as they have less reserve than adults so that there is more potential for harm. Doctors hold several concerns about complementary or alternative therapies. Many of the therapies have no scientific basis, and the way they are supposed to work is not consistent with our understanding of how the body works. There are many examples of serious illness and even occasional deaths caused by the ingredients in so-called 'natural' therapies. Patients are given some mixture of tablets of so-called natural ingredients, but they contain substances that may be harmful if taken in high doses, or can cause an allergic reaction in some individuals, or else react with other medicines the person is taking. The potential for a dangerous situation arising in young children is greater because of their lower reserve. Finally, there is the concern that relying on natural therapies and natural treatments may postpone the early diagnosis and implementation of an effective treatment for serious illnesses.

Often parents seek alternative or natural therapies for their children because they do not like the idea of giving medicines to their children. They think somehow that medicines weaken the immune system or poison the body. While in a number of conditions medicines are unnecessary and generally prescribed too freely, in other conditions they are life saving. It should also be borne in mind that just because medicines are 'natural' does not mean that they are better or less harmful to the body. Some of the so-called natural remedies in fact have very high concentrations of pharmacological ingredients in them.

The challenge for all of us is to keep an open mind about complementary medicines and therapies while at the same time recognising that some therapies are unlikely to be of benefit and can even be harmful. The first port of call for childhood illness should always be the general practitioner. It is important that professional staff looking after children, whatever the setting, be aware of any medicines or alternate therapies that the child is taking or using. Any type of medication should always be taken in accordance with the instructions.

Television

Children are usually first exposed to television (TV) as early as infancy. By the time they begin preschool, they will likely recognise TV characters and have their favourite programs. TV has become an important part of the lives of most children. Some TV can be very beneficial — there are some very good educational and other child-oriented programs, and some excellent children's videos. They should not be regarded as a substitute for reading or playing, but TV can be the child's first exposure to colours and numbers and a whole range of positive experiences that can stimulate and challenge them. But for all the potential benefits of TV to children, there are also major problems with children watching TV.

Research suggests that the average child spends more time each year watching TV than going to school. These TV watching habits begin earlier in life. TV, therefore, can have a pervasive effect on the lives of children. Whether this turns out to be beneficial or harmful is largely under the control of parents. While early childhood professionals cannot be expected to be responsible for the TV watching habits of the children in their care, nevertheless, because of their trusted role with parents, they can be influential in helping parents understand the harmful effects of TV.

There is a strong link between the amount of time spent watching TV and obesity. Children who watch a lot of TV are less active and are more likely to snack while watching. 'Junk foods' are often advertised at times when children are likely to be watching, as are toys that encourage violent behaviour. There is a well-established association between aggressive behaviour in young children and them having seen violence on TV. Young children are unable to differentiate fantasy from fact. If they see violence and aggression on the screen, they may come to think that this is normal and even desirable behaviour. There is much stereotyping of characters on TV still, whether it is women or people from certain cultural or ethnic backgrounds.

Watching TV is mostly passive and, while children can learn from it, there are other activities which offer much richer learning experiences that will enhance the child's natural curiosity and creativity. One of the best things that one can do for young children is to turn off the TV. Early childhood professionals can help parents understand how to make the TV set a positive experience for their child. They can suggest that parents actively select programs for their child to watch, rather than have the TV on all the time by default, to limit the time the child watches TV, and to be conscious of the time where the TV is used as a distraction or as a passive babysitter.

Computer games

Like television, computer games have the potential to be of immense benefit to young children and also the capacity to be harmful. There is an increasing number of very good educational games that are suitable for children from the older toddler-age period upwards. Carefully chosen, these can provide wonderful creative entertainment and, unlike television, the child is involved as an active participant. In theory, they have the capacity to promote activities that may influence aspects of the child's development and cognitive functioning, like eye-hand coordination and letter and number recognition. However, there is no evidence that these educational games make any difference to intelligence or improve developmental functioning. There are claims made for some games that they will enhance development or turn the young child into an early and fluent reader. These claims should be treated with caution.

On the downside are those games that have themes of violence or aggression. There is a growing body of evidence pointing to the harmful effects of having young children exposed to violence or aggressive behaviour, whether this is in real life, movies or cartoons, or computer games. Early childhood professionals are in a unique position to give guidance to parents on these issues.

Reading/literacy

Being able to read well is one of the most important attributes anyone can have in life. Reading ability is a major predictor of school success and, therefore, of self-confidence and self-esteem. The reverse is also true. Reading difficulties are a major barrier to a successful and productive life.

Research shows that one of the most important pointers to reading success is whether a child was exposed to books from a young age. Those who are read to as young children — from as young as six months of age — are more likely to come to enjoy books and reading and to become successful readers. It follows then that reading to their young child is one of the most important activities that parents can undertake. At six months, infants will simply enjoy the sound of their parents' voice and being held in a position where they can see the images and pictures in the book. As they get older, they will reach out and want to turn pages. Their concentration span may be short initially, but with increasing age and maturity they will be able to focus better. Many parents are amazed at how quiet and enthralled their toddler becomes when read to. As their language and cognitive ability increases, they will begin to listen to the content of the story, and soon will be able to recognise and point to the pictures. Before long they will begin to read their own book, initially in a make-believe manner as they will not be able to really read.

However they will come to know the pleasure of sitting on their parents' lap and hearing their voice and looking at a book. Soon they will come to associate books with stories, and then associate letters and words written on the page with meaning. Acquiring this level of interest in books and reading means that they are off to a great start in achieving literacy; these pre-literacy skills usually translate into good literacy skills.

Early childhood professionals should do all they can to promote reading to young children. In addition to making it one of the central activities they undertake with children in their care, they are in a unique position to share this conviction with parents. Talking to parents about the importance of reading, suggesting age and developmentally appropriate books that they can buy, reminding them that it is never too early for their young child to join the local library, modelling reading behaviours for the parents — these are all ways in which professionals can help parents develop a passion about reading to their young child, which then creates the best possible opportunity for the child to grow up passionate about reading. There is almost nothing we can do for young children that is more worthwhile.

Smoking

The health risks associated with smoking have been well known to health professionals for a long time. Now communities are accepting more stringent laws about smoking in public places. Apart from the health hazards for the smokers themselves, there are also risks to non-smokers from 'passive smoking' — inhaling cigarette smoke because they are in the vicinity of smokers.

No child should be exposed to cigarette smoke, even in utero. Babies born to mothers who smoke during pregnancy are much more likely to be small and have a low birth weight. There is research linking the onset of asthma to exposure to cigarette smoke early in life. Parental smoking is one of the risk factors for Sudden Infant Death Syndrome (SIDS). Exposure to cigarette smoke worsens any respiratory conditions in children — it can trigger an attack of asthma and young children whose parents smoke have a higher incidence of bronchiolitis and pneumonia . . . the list goes on and on.

All places where children play or learn or are cared for should be smoke-free. Professionals working with children can also encourage parents either to quit smoking themselves, or at least to make sure that their children are reared in smoke-free environments.

The link between illness and behaviour

Young children always provide important clues as to how sick they are by their behaviour. As long as they are behaving fairly normally then, whatever the condition or the illness that is causing the child's symptoms, it is unlikely to be serious. The more normal the child's behaviour is, the more likely is it that the illness is minor and not serious. The converse is also true. The more the child's behaviour is different from how she normally is, the more likely it is that the illness may be serious.

This is further discussed in the section on fever (page 38). The fever itself, even if it is high, is not a concern in and of itself. Rather, it is the behaviour of the child that provides the most important clue as to how serious the illness is. The child who continues to be interested in her surroundings, in interacting with other children and with carers or teachers, who wants to take part in activities and play, who can still smile or laugh, is unlikely to have an illness that is a major cause for worry.

2

Immunisation and Infection Control

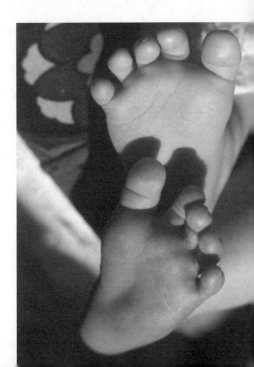

As young children begin to have contact with the wider world — attending playgroup, family day care, child care, preschool — it is inevitable that they will be exposed to viruses and bacteria that cause a range of infections. Most of these thankfully are not serious — colds and upper respiratory infections and other viral infections are part and parcel of growing up.

Infection can be spread in several ways. The most common is from person to person. A child or adult may have an active infection or is incubating an infection which is not yet apparent, and inadvertently spreads it to others with whom he comes into contact. The infection can be spread in a number of ways.

▶ Droplet spread, by coughing or sneezing — This is the commonest way that colds and upper respiratory infections are spread, especially in winter when people tend to be in close contact in confined spaces.

▶ Direct contact, either from person to person or with infected surfaces — This is why washing of hands is so important after changing a nappy or wiping a child's runny nose. Also important in preventing the spread of infections is washing toys and utensils that are shared by young children, properly wiping down benches and tabletops, and properly disposing of soiled nappies or tissues.

While it is impossible to completely prevent the spread of infection, there are effective measures that can be taken to minimise infections in settings where children congregate. All child-care centres and preschools operate within the framework of government regulations and there are accreditation guidelines that address infection control. There are many effective precautions and measures that can be taken to prevent the spread of infection. Research has shown that where these are implemented, there is often a dramatic reduction in infection. A detailed teaching package on prevention of infection has been developed and is distributed at nominal cost by the Centre for Community Child Health in Melbourne. It consists of a video, professional workbook and posters, and can be obtained by calling (03) 9345 6150, or sending an email to <enquiries.ccch@rch.org.au>.

Each state also has health regulations that govern the exclusion of children who have specified infectious diseases; these vary from state to state. Information can be obtained by contacting the local health department.

Finally the National Childcare Accreditation Council (NCAC) accreditation guidelines include an emphasis on hygiene and infection control. These guidelines are intended to set national 'best practice' standards to protect the health of young children and protect their wellbeing. They suggest that each child-care centre and family-day care centre refer to the appropriate health authorities in each state/territory to ensure they comply with regulations for hygiene and infection control. Details of the accreditation guidelines are available from the NCAC office in Sydney:

National Childcare Accreditation Council, Level 3, 418A Elizabeth Street, Surry Hills NSW 2010, Phone (02) 8260 1900 or 1300 136 554, Fax (02) 8260 1901, Email: qualitycare@ncac.gov.au; Internet <http://www.ncac.gov.au>.

Immunisation

Immunisation is just about the most effective of all strategies designed to protect the health of young children. All children should be fully immunised. Checking immunisation status and ensuring full immunisation is an important responsibility of those working in community settings with young children.

The way immunisation works is that a killed or weakened strain of a germ (virus or bacteria) is given to the child (or adult), either by mouth or injection. This causes the body's immune system to make antibodies to that particular disease; antibodies recognise and fight the real and active viruses or bacteria when the child is exposed to them. There are vaccines which protect against a number of very serious and potentially fatal diseases, and there are new vaccines being introduced from time to time.

Currently children in Australia are immunised against the following infectious diseases:

▶ diphtheria;
▶ measles;
▶ mumps;
▶ rubella (German measles);
▶ tetanus;
▶ pertussis (whooping cough);
▶ polio;
▶ haemophilus B (HIB);
▶ hepatitis B; and
▶ meningococcus.

From 2003, all children who turn 12 months and all preschool children aged 1–5 years are eligible for meningococcus vaccines.

There are other recommended vaccines which are now available, though at the time of writing they are not yet on the schedule for all children. These include:

▶ pneumococcus (causes pneumonia, blood infections, meningitis and ear infections);
▶ varicella (chicken pox); and
▶ influenza.

Parents should be encouraged especially to have their child immunised against pneumococcus, which can cause serious infections.

This list of conditions is current at the time of writing, but is being added to on a regular basis as new vaccines become available. The current schedule is available at

<**http://immunise.health.gov.au/schedule**>. See below for ways in which information about the current schedule can be obtained. Further information and any needed clarification can also be obtained from a GP or paediatrician.

Due to the success of immunisation programs, many of these conditions are rarely seen today. This has led to a sense of complacency in some sections of the community. One only has to talk to some of the older doctors or to grandparents who have vivid memories still of polio epidemics or hospital wards full of children with diphtheria. And it is only recently that children were fighting for their lives because of haemophilus influenza infections, which caused the very serious and potentially fatal epiglottitis and meningitis.

Apart from the clear benefits of immunisation for each individual child, it is also important from a community view that all children are immunised. As well as being at greater risk of contracting these infections, non-immunised children also help spread infection in the community.

Despite it being the single most effective public health measure for children, some parents still hold reservations about immunising their children, and there are still misconceptions about different aspects of immunisation. Non-health professionals cannot be expected to engage in discussions with parents about detailed aspects of immunisation programs — they should be encouraged to speak to the child's doctor or community nurse about these, or there is information available from the state and commonwealth health departments. But it is reasonable to expect all professionals who come into contact with children and their parents to check on immunisation status and make sure that all children in their care are fully immunised.

Immunisation schedule

Outlined below is the current immunisation schedule for Australian children as recommended by the National Health and Medical Research Council (NHMRC), which is the government body responsible for reviewing and updating the schedule as new vaccines become available. This is up to date at the time this book goes to press, but is likely to be changed as new vaccines become available. It is also likely that the number of injections will be reduced, as some vaccines will be able to be combined into a single injection. There is also research looking at other ways of children receiving immunisation, such as by mouth or via nasal drops or spray. The local doctor, community nurse, or state or commonwealth health department can always provide you with a current schedule. You can also check the current immunisation schedule on the website of the NHMRC. The schedule can be found at <**http://immunise.health.gov.au/schedule**>.

Age	Vaccine
Birth	Hepatitis B
2 months	Diphtheria Pertussis Tetanus Polio Haemophilus influenzae Hepatitis B
4 months	Diphtheria Pertussis Tetanus Polio Haemophilus influenzae Hepatitis B
6 months	Diphtheria Pertussis Tetanus Polio Hepatitis B (some schedules omit this at this age)
12 months*	Measles Mumps Rubella Haemophilus influenzae Hepatitis B (if not given at 6 months)
18 months*	Diphtheria Pertussis Tetanus
4 years*	Diphtheria Pertussis Tetanus Measles Mumps Rubella Polio

* Meningococcus is available from 12 months (single injection).

Reactions to immunisation

Immunisations are not totally without side effects. Many children will have a reaction following immunisation; these are nearly always minor and transient. The most common, perhaps inevitable, is the child's reaction to the pain of the injection. This can be minimised by giving paracetamol beforehand, by having the parent hold the child during the injection and cuddle her immediately afterwards, and by offering the breast or a bottle or pacifier for the child to suck on.

Many children may have swelling and redness at the injection site; some have a mild fever. Parents may report that their child is irritable or not hungry or 'not herself'. These reactions are usually mild and last anywhere from a few hours to a few days; they can be minimised by giving paracetamol immediately before and then for 24 hours following immunisation.

Serious reactions are rare. The child is at far greater risk of harm (or even death) from contracting one of the infections because she is not immunised than from the immunisation itself.

3

Children's Health in Practice

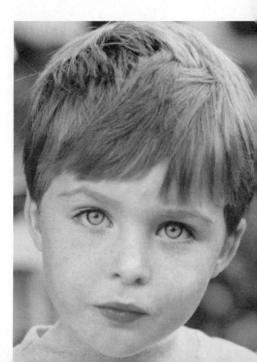

First aid kit

Every early childhood setting should have a well-stocked, well-maintained first aid kit. This should not be used as an alternative to timely medical advice. Rather, it is for use in emergencies until medical assistance can be obtained, or for the treatment of simple problems. The first aid kit should be kept in a clearly marked and locked place and all staff should be able to access it when needed. There should be a protocol in place so it is checked on a regular basis and items replaced as they are used or as they pass their expiry date. It is also possible to buy commercial first aid kits of varying sizes.

The following contents of a first aid kit are recommended as a minimum:

▶ adhesive tape — preferably in several different widths;
▶ alcohol wipes;
▶ bandages (crepe) of various sizes — at least 3 of each width;
▶ bandaids of various shapes and sizes — several packets;
▶ cotton wool balls;
▶ disinfectant;
▶ dressings (sterile and non-stick) — a number of different sizes;
▶ eye pads (sterile);
▶ gauze (sterile) — several packets;
▶ gloves (disposable latex);
▶ needle (to remove splinters);
▶ pocket first aid book;
▶ safety pins;
▶ scissors;
▶ sling;
▶ steristrips (sterile) for closing small cuts;
▶ thermometer; and
▶ tweezers.

In addition, a medicine kit can be put together and contain the following:

▶ antihistamine (for allergic reactions);
▶ antiseptic solution (iodine);
▶ calamine lotion;
▶ measuring cup (for medicine); and
▶ paracetamol.

It is also useful to include such items as sunscreen, insect repellent, and nappy rash cream, as well as emergency contact numbers — ambulance, police, fire brigade, poisons information centre, local hospital, local GP and community nurse, and any other useful numbers. These should also be prominently displayed in other places, such as next to the telephone.

Emergencies

Ideally, all children's settings should have a handbook on first aid, a comprehensive first aid kit, at least one member of staff trained in first aid and preferably cardiopulmonary resuscitation (CPR), guidelines about what to do in particular emergencies, and an easily accessible list of emergency phone numbers — these should include ambulance, police, fire brigade, poisons information service, hospital, and nearest doctor.

In an urgent situation the following action should be undertaken, *in this order*:

1. Remove the child from immediate danger.

2. Think ABC

   Airway — Make sure the child has a clear and unobstructed airway. Place the child on his side with his head back and his chin tilted upwards. Clear the mouth of any food.

   Breathing — Check that the child is breathing. If not, begin cardiopulmonary resuscitation, as demonstrated in the first aid book.

   Circulation — Make sure that the child has a pulse. If not, then commence cardiopulmonary resuscitation.

3. Treat any severe bleeding.

4. Treat any severe burns.

5. Seek medical assistance at the first opportunity.

If you are alone, urgent first aid is a priority before you call for help. If others are present, someone should be delegated to seek medical assistance.

Allergic reactions

True allergies are relatively uncommon in children, though many symptoms ranging from infant crying to rashes to diarrhoea are sometimes wrongly attributed to allergy. However, there is a very small number of children who have a genuine very severe allergy, usually to a food such as peanuts or shellfish, to medicines such as penicillin, or sometimes to a bee sting or insect bite. The reaction varies in severity, but in its severest form (anaphylactic shock, see below) can be life threatening.

Milder cases of acute allergy can result in puffy eyes, an itchy rash or swelling of parts of the body. In more serious cases, the swelling of face and eyes is more rapid and extensive, and the child may have difficulty breathing because the throat, voice box and windpipe are involved. In the most severe cases of allergic reaction, the child becomes pale and clammy, with great difficulty in breathing.

It is important at the time of enrolment at the early childhood setting to check for any history of allergies — prevention is always the best option. Where an allergic reaction has occurred, seek *immediate* medical help. *In the unlikely event of unexpected anaphylactic shock, call for an ambulance immediately.*

Those children who have been identified as having severe allergies will often have an emergency kit near them — parents will always make sure it is in the car or at home, and will arrange for the early childhood setting to have it available for use in emergencies. Such a kit consists of an adrenaline injection, and clearly parents will have to have given very clear instructions of when and how to use it.

Bites and stings

Bee stings

Most bee stings cause pain, swelling and itch. The bee sting has a barb on the end so it stays in the skin together with the sac of venom. This should be carefully removed with a fingernail, making sure that the skin is *not* squeezed. Scraping action with the fingernail is the most effective way of removing the sting. Applying an ice pack that is wrapped first in a tea towel or cloth may be soothing and help to reduce the swelling, and then application of calamine lotion is a time-honoured and partially effective treatment. The swelling reduces after a day or two, and the itch and pain also rapidly resolve.

A small number of children are highly allergic to bee stings, in which case special precautions need to be taken and emergency treatment instituted (see Allergic reactions, page 18).

Dog bites

Young children and dogs are a potentially dangerous combination. The natural enthusiasm, curiosity and quick, unpredictable movements of toddlers and preschoolers means that they are at risk of being bitten by dogs, who react instinctively. The bite may range from a trivial graze where the skin is barely broken through to severe lacerations and injuries sometimes needing admission to hospital for surgery.

Treatment depends on the extent of the injury. The child will invariably be frightened and traumatised by the bite, and needs to be held and comforted. Dog saliva carries many germs; if the skin is broken then the child needs to have a course of antibiotics to make sure that the bite does not become infected. If the skin is broken, the child should be seen by a doctor as soon as possible so that immunisation status can be checked (the child's tetanus protection needs to be confirmed), antibiotics prescribed, and the bite assessed.

Mosquito bites

Mosquitoes are prominent during the summer months, and bites occur mainly at dusk and in the evening. They cause itchy red swellings, worse in some children who seem more sensitive to mosquito bites. If the symptoms are very troublesome, an ice pack that is wrapped first in a tea towel or cloth can help reduce the swelling, and calamine lotion can be applied to reduce the itch. Children should be discouraged from scratching at the bites, as they can become infected. Taking precautions to prevent mosquito bites is a good idea. The application of a simple insect repellent, preferably a roll-on for young children, should be considered when young children are likely to be exposed to mosquito bites.

Snake bites

Not all snakes in Australia are venomous, but a bite from one that is venomous can be lethal and urgent action must be taken immediately. Try to identify the snake if possible. As identification is sometimes difficult, any snake bite must be considered potentially very serious and a medical emergency. Keep the child as still and quiet as possible. Do not wash the wound or cut it, and do not try to suck the venom out. Immediately apply a pressure immobilisation bandage (see below), elevate the limb, and call an ambulance or take the child to the nearest hospital as it is more likely than the general practitioner to carry supplies of the antivenom. Most regional hospitals will be aware of the snakes in that area and will carry the appropriate antivenom.

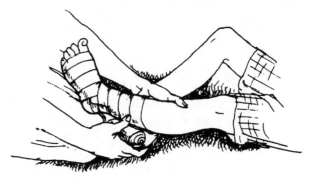

A *pressure immobilisation bandage* is considered the most appropriate initial treatment for snake bite or spider bite. Keep the bitten area still. Do not remove clothing as the movement of the limb while doing this will help to spread the venom in the body. Apply a wide crepe bandage. If a bandage is not immediately available, strips of material or a tea towel can be used. The bandage should be tight enough to exert a firm pressure on the limb, but not that tight that it cuts off the circulation. Extend the bandage as far as possible on either side of the bite, beginning at the end of the limb and working upwards. For example, if the bite is on the ankle, begin at the toes and bandage right up to the thigh. Then tie a splint to the limb; anything will do — a cricket bat, a fence paling, or a broomstick. If the bite is on the arm a sling will keep the arm from moving too much. Then seek medical help as a matter of urgency.

Spider bites

There are two types of spiders in Australia whose bites can be lethal — the funnel-web and the red-back. The funnel-web is found mostly in New South Wales, while the red-back can be found throughout Australia.

If it is suspected that the bite is from one of these two spiders, consider this a medical emergency. Apply a pressure immobilisation bandage over the bite. Then, either call an ambulance or take the child immediately to the nearest hospital. If the spider is dead try to take it with you for identification.

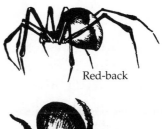

Red-back

A *pressure immobilisation bandage* is a wide crepe bandage. If a bandage is not immediately available, strips of material or a tea towel can be used. The bandage should be tight enough to exert a firm pressure on the limb, but not that tight that it cuts off the circulation. Extend

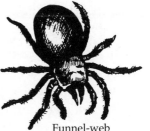

Funnel-web

the bandage as far as possible on either side of the bite, beginning at the end of the limb and working upwards. For example, if the bite is on the ankle, begin at the toes and bandage right up to the thigh. Then tie a splint to the limb; anything will do — a cricket bat, a fence paling, or a broomstick. If the bite is on the arm, a sling will keep the arm from moving too much. Then seek medical help as a matter of urgency.

However any spider bite, even if it is not dangerous, can be very painful and cause local swelling and discomfort. If the pain persists or there is local bruising, then it is safest to seek medical advice.

Wasp stings

Wasps can inflict multiple stings; these can be painful and cause considerable swelling around the stings. An ice pack that is wrapped first in a tea towel or cloth can reduce the amount of swelling and discomfort. Care should be taken drinking directly from a can of soft drink when outdoors. Wasps are attracted to the sugar and can enter the can.

Bleeding

The most common causes of bleeding are cuts and abrasions. In the course of everyday exploration, most children at some stage or another will experience some sort of trauma that will result in a cut or abrasion. It may be because of a fall, or cutting themselves on a sharp object, or physical contact with another child. Thankfully, most of these are not serious though, of course, they cause pain and distress to the child.

In an abrasion, blood oozes slowly and unevenly from the skin surface as the very small vessels in the skin have been damaged. This bleeding is easy to stop with gentle but firm pressure for a minute or two. Wash the abrasion with warm water and soap, gently brushing away any dirt or foreign material. Sometimes this is all that is necessary. If the abrasion is large, or there has been some persistent ooze, then it is best to cover it with sterile gauze. Antiseptic cream can also be applied, though this is not essential.

A scratch or cut can also cause bleeding. If it is small, with the skin surface broken only superficially, then pressure over the cut should quickly stop the bleeding. Washing it and then applying a bandaid is all that is needed. Some cuts are deeper and the edges are gaping. Sometimes the bleeding is profuse. Cuts to the head or scalp are especially prone to bleed a lot because of the rich blood supply to these areas.

The best way to stop the bleeding is to apply firm pressure over the site of the bleeding. In time, the body's natural clotting mechanism kicks in and the bleeding will stop. This usually takes only a minute or two. Where bleeding is profuse or persistent, it is always a good idea to seek medical attention as sutures (stitches) may be required.

Very occasionally the bleeding may be spurting in quality and a bright red in colour, rather than the darker red of simple cuts. This suggests that a small artery has been severed. Again, this is treated with firm and persistent pressure, the limb raised if the cut is on the arm or leg, and urgent medical attention sought. Pressure is best applied with gauze or, in an emergency, with a clean towel or any material that is handy.

When dealing with any bleeding wound, it is essential that latex or plastic gloves are worn, and that all blood-stained materials be placed in a plastic bag which is then sealed and disposed of properly. Any bloody surfaces should be washed down with hot water and soap and then cleaned thoroughly with a disinfectant. In this way, the chances of blood-borne cross-infection are minimised.

Bleeding from the mouth

Injuries to the mouth usually bleed profusely because of the rich blood supply to this area. The bleeding can be from a split lip, a lacerated tongue, a tooth through the lip, or from tooth damage. If possible, apply pressure to the bleeding area, and seek medical help as soon as possible.

Bleeding from the nose

This can occur either from a blow to the nose as the result of a fall or other trauma, or from blowing or picking the nose, or may occur spontaneously in association with a cold. The bleeding stems from tiny capillaries in the nasal septum and is rarely serious. It can be just a small amount on a tissue or handkerchief that appears when the child blows his nose, in which case nothing needs to be done. Sometimes there is a small amount of bleeding from a nostril that stops quickly if the child sits quietly. Often gentle pressure on the side of the nose will help. On occasion, the bleeding is more profuse and then it is best to pinch both nostrils for a few minutes with the child leaning forward.

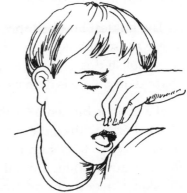

The child may become distressed by the bleeding, and may gag because the blood from the nose is swallowed. If the bleeding occurs frequently, the child should see a doctor who may cauterise the affected blood vessels in the nose.

Burns and scalds

Burns may be caused by contact with hot objects, fire, or friction. Scalds are caused by hot water or steam. They can vary in severity from minor burns or scalds that need no active treatment to those severe enough to require hospitalisation and that can endanger life.

The mildest burns simply cause the skin to go red, even though they can be painful. These are sometimes called first-degree burns. The next level of severity is when it causes blistering of the skin, and the most severe is when the skin looks almost white or charred and there is damage to the whole thickness of the skin.

If a child is burned or scalded, immediately rinse the affected area with cold water to cool the area and relieve the pain — two to three minutes is enough. Do *not* use ice. Remove any clothing from the burnt area unless it is stuck to the skin. Cover the burnt area with a sterile gauze and seek medical attention.

Do not pierce any blisters or cut away any peeling skin. *Never* put butter or grease or powder on a burn, in fact it is best to avoid putting on any creams or lotions until after the child has had a medical assessment.

All burns and scalds are, theoretically, preventable. Regulations about fire protection, including smoke detectors and appropriate safeguards on heaters and fireplaces, are very strict and should be obeyed to the letter. Always be very careful with hot liquids, whether it is boiling water in an electric kettle or urn or on the stove, or in the form of a cup of tea or coffee in the hands of an adult. Remember that curious toddlers can easily pull at the edge of a tablecloth and pull down hot liquids which appear to be out of reach. Hot water systems should be adjusted by a plumber so that the water is at a temperature that cannot scald a child.

Choking

All infants and young toddlers put things in their mouth; this is part of their exploration and learning at this age. This should always be kept in mind when selecting toys; make sure that there are no small bits that young children can swallow or inhale. Young children should always be seated when eating, and care taken with food selection. Peanuts are best avoided completely in preschool children and hard foods, such as carrots, best avoided or else given under close supervision.

The child who is choking may begin to cough or splutter, and may turn blue. Immediately tip the child head down so that the coughing may dislodge the object. Slap the child firmly on the back between the shoulder blades, and call for medical assistance.

Convulsions and epilepsy (fits, seizures)

Convulsions can occur in a number of circumstances in young children. Most commonly they may be associated with a fever, and are called febrile convulsions. These last for a few seconds to a minute or two at the most and, although frightening to witness, do not result in any long-term problems. In particular, a febrile convulsion does not mean the child has or will go on to develop a seizure disorder. Some children do have epilepsy, and despite the very good treatments available designed to prevent seizures, may still have them from time to time. This information should be obtained from parents when a health profile is created at the time of enrolment.

Most seizures occur without warning, though in some forms of epilepsy there is an aura (like a premonition). Most young children, however, will not be aware of this. The child may fall to the ground, her body will stiffen and jerk uncontrollably, the eyes will roll into the back of her head, and the teeth will be clenched. Sometimes there will be frothing of the mouth, and the child may wet or soil herself. Usually it will not last for more than a few minutes at the most, or considerably shorter, though occasionally a child may have a prolonged seizure. Immediately afterwards the child will be drowsy and want to sleep.

When the seizure is actually taking place, there are a number of things a bystander can do:

▶ Remain calm — this is very important.

▶ Loosen the child's clothes and remove eye glasses.

▶ Move objects and furniture away to make sure the child cannot injure herself.

▶ Position her onto her side so she is less likely to swallow her tongue or any vomit in case she is sick.

▶ Allow her to move freely – do not attempt to restrain her.

▶ Do not force anything into her mouth.

▶ After the seizure has finished, lay her on her side and allow her to sleep.

▶ Do not give any food or drink until she is fully awake.

▶ If the seizure lasts longer than five minutes, seek medical help urgently — call an ambulance.

▶ Change any wet or soiled clothes.

▶ The child should be seen by a doctor as soon as possible the same day.

Drowning

Young children have no sense of the danger of water and their natural curiosity places them in danger. Children drown either because they get into water that is too deep, or else they get trapped while their faces are submerged. They can drown even in very shallow amounts of water only a few centimetres deep. If a child is found in water, think ABC (see page 17). Begin resuscitation immediately if he is not breathing, and call for medical assistance. Children need to be supervised at all times around water, whether it is in the bath, around a pool, at the sea or by a river or dam. Never leave even a bucket of water standing where young children can get to it. Empty water from sinks, and empty or cover wading pools when not in use.

Foreign bodies

Children are always putting objects into places where they should not go — into ears, up their nose, or swallowing them. It is difficult to prevent them doing this; it is part of their curiosity.

Ear

The foreign body can be almost anything, ranging from a small bead or part of a toy through to a pea or small stone. Sometimes an insect finds its way into the child's ear. The child is usually aware of the presence of the foreign body in the ear, and will draw attention to it. Sometimes it is right on the edge of the ear, and a piece can be grabbed onto easily and the whole object pulled out. However, often it is a smooth, round object that is deeply lodged in the ear, and then the child needs to be taken to the doctor or hospital for removal.

Nose

Usually the child draws attention that something is stuck in her nose, but occasionally the child is not aware or has forgotten about it. In these cases one nostril can be obstructed to breathing, or there can be bleeding or a discharge from one nostril. In virtually all cases, the child needs to be taken to the doctor or hospital for removal of the object.

Mouth

Young children can swallow anything — beads, coins, bits of toys, buttons, and even sometimes safety pins. Mostly they pass without any great difficulty, especially if they are small and round. Sharp objects, such as pins or pieces of glass, may be more problematic. It is always a good idea to have the child checked by a doctor. If the object is small and smooth, it will certainly pass through the child's intestine within a couple of days and be seen in a bowel motion. If it is larger, an X-ray may be called for to check that it has passed through the gullet into the stomach. If this is the case, then it will pass safely; the junction between the gullet and stomach is the narrowest part of the gastro-intestinal tract. If the object is sharp, there is a very good chance that it will need to be removed in hospital.

Eye

Everybody has had the problem of a foreign body in the eye. This can be an eyelash or a foreign body such as a speck of sand or dirt, and this is common in young children too. The eye will be painful, watery, and will soon become bloodshot. The usual tendency will be to rub the eye, but often this will make it worse and should be discouraged. Sometimes the foreign body is visible and can be removed with the edge of a clean handkerchief or tissue. Check the lower lid by gently pulling the lid downwards or the upper lid by inverting it over a cotton bud or match. If the particle is visible, very gently try to remove it. If it is hard to remove, or if the particle cannot be seen, then it is best to have the child seen by a doctor.

Fractures and dislocations

A fracture (broken bone) is the result of considerable trauma, usually the result of a fall or collision or other accident. The pain is severe and the affected part quickly becomes swollen, with limited and very painful movement, and sometimes a visible deformity. Depending on the incident, there may be other internal injuries as well, so a doctor should always see the child as soon as possible.

Immediate management depends on the body part that is fractured. Occasionally the skin is broken with visible external bleeding and perhaps even the bone visible. Make the child as comfortable as possible by minimising the amount of movement of the affected part. The arm can be immobilised by a splint or sling, while a splint can be fashioned to keep a broken leg still.

With a dislocation, bony parts are pushed out of alignment due to stretching of the ligaments as a result of trauma. The immediate management is the same as for a fracture — immobilise the part and have the child seen by a doctor as soon as possible.

Head injuries

Head injuries can be trivial or serious and life threatening, and it is not always easy to be sure of the severity as sometimes manifestations may not become apparent until hours or days afterwards. A head injury can result in loss of consciousness, or else there can be no apparent immediate consequences. There may be bruising or abrasion or a cut — these should be treated appropriately (see Bleeding, page 22).

If the child has suffered a severe blow to the head, it is always a good idea to seek early medical advice. Immediately after the injury, make sure the child is breathing properly, and lie him on his side. Allow him to get up and move around if he wishes. If *any* of the following occurs in association with a head injury, then urgent medical assessment is required:

- loss of consciousness;
- unequal pupils or eyes that are bloodshot;
- any fluid, clear or bloodstained, coming from the nose or ears;
- convulsions;
- drowsiness, confusion or loss of memory;
- persistent headache;
- nausea or vomiting; and
- unsteadiness in walking, or any other unusual symptoms.

Poisoning

Ingested

Sometimes it will be obvious that the child has swallowed poison — someone may see him drink or eat poisonous substances, or else the child may be discovered with an open or empty container of tablets or medicine or a toxic substance. Also think of poisoning if there are burn marks on his lips or mouth, if there are unexplained stains on his clothing and he has an unusual odour about him, if he is drooling or has unexplained nausea or vomiting, or any changes in his behaviour such as irritability or drowsiness.

The treatment depends on the type of poison ingested. Do not induce vomiting — this is not necessarily the best treatment unless it is immediately after an ingestion, and for some poisons inducing vomiting is dangerous. Contact the poisons information centre (the phone number should be displayed in a prominent place, along with other emergency numbers) and follow their advice. They will want to know what the child has ingested, as well as his age and weight if it is available, and the time when it was ingested.

On the skin

If the child spills a dangerous substance onto his skin, remove his clothes and rinse the area with warm water. If the area shows signs of being burned, continue to rinse with water for 5–10 minutes. Do *not* apply creams or any other substance. Call the poisons information centre for further advice.

In the eye

Flush the child's eye by holding his eyelid open and pouring a stream of lukewarm water into the inner corner of the eye. Using a jug is best. Continue this for 5–10 minutes. Get somebody to hold the child or else wrap his arms by his sides using a towel. Then seek medical advice.

Injury prevention

Injuries are the commonest cause of death in childhood after the first year of life, and a major reason for a child being admitted to hospital or needing medical attention. Most injuries in young children do not occur by chance or by bad luck; they are predictable and largely preventable. Safety issues form a major part of the regulations for agencies and places in the community where there are young children, and are also a key component of the accreditation system for child care and family day care. Nevertheless, all adults who have a responsibility for young children owe it to them and to their parents to make absolutely certain that the places where children congregate are as safe as they can possibly be.

This pertains both to the physical surroundings and to the day-to-day functioning. Make sure the environment is safe — sturdy toys that do not have small parts that can be detached and inhaled or swallowed; safe play equipment with soft surfaces underneath; shaded areas for sun protection; dangerous substances stored well away and preferably in childproof cupboards or under lock and key; plugs on power points and short or curly cords on electrical appliances; guards in front of fires and heaters; furniture that is appropriate to the age of the children and which does not have sharp corners; safety barriers at the top and bottom of stairs; the list goes on. Many issues need to be kept in mind if injuries are to be prevented. These include the level of training and knowledge of staff about child development and expectations and capabilities of each age group; the level of supervision of children's play and activities; the ratios of staff to children to allow adequate supervision; the range of toys and equipment used in day-to-day activities; the safety of the environment — surfaces, separation from traffic and other potential hazards.

Young children are by their very nature active, curious, impulsive, excitable — all qualities that make them vulnerable to injuring themselves. We cannot and should not try to change the children. Rather it is their environment that we need to make safe for them. On the other hand, there are numerous opportunities for early childhood professionals to teach children safety issues in the course of normal day-to-day activities — not running across a car park, crossing roads where there are traffic lights or supervised crossings, teaching about car restraints, and so on.

In addition to providing a safe environment for children in early childhood settings, this can also provide important modelling for parents. The relationship an early childhood professional has with parents creates the opportunity to talk to them not only about the emerging abilities and social competencies of their children, but also about how their rapid development and natural curiosity makes it essential that they pay attention to safety issues at home and while travelling.

Further information about child safety and safety standards can be obtained from Kidsafe, a national organisation with branches in each state which are usually attached to the children's hospitals in each capital city or, in Victoria, from the Safety Centre at the Royal Children's Hospital.

The sick baby and child
Recognising serious illness in infants and young children

No child enjoys perfect health all of the time. The most common illnesses are the common viral infections that every child contracts, especially in the winter months, and which are more common in those who attend child care or preschool. There are many other illnesses and conditions of childhood that are described in this book. Some are serious and require specialist care and treatment; others are not of great concern and get better quickly without any special treatment.

However, even illnesses which are usually benign and self-limiting sometimes are more serious and need accurate diagnosis and specific medical treatment. The early childhood professional sometimes has to deal with a child who is unwell. In most instances the parent will be notified and appropriate action taken, such as seeking medical advice. In some instances there may be a delay in being able to contact parents.

Every early childhood setting and community agency that looks after young children should have clearly established guidelines for the management of medical emergencies and illness in children, and should also have an established relationship with a local doctor who can readily provide advice or attend if needed. The local doctor can help with the development of guidelines that are relevant and appropriate for the specific setting.

However it is useful for early childhood professionals to have some understanding of the signs and symptoms that suggest that a young child may be quite sick and need urgent medical attention. These include:

▶ High fever: A high fever in a young child is a sign of infection and needs to be investigated to find the cause. However fever by itself is not necessarily an indicator of serious illness (see below, page 38).

▶ Drowsiness: Note whether the infant or young child is less alert than normal, making less eye contact, and less interested in her surroundings.

▶ Lethargy and decreased activity: The child wants to lie down or be held rather than participate in any activity, even those that normally would have been of interest.

▶ Breathing difficulty: This is an important sign. She may be breathing very quickly, or the breathing may be very noisy, or she may be fighting hard to get a breath. She may be coughing, or be blue around the mouth. She may be working hard at breathing, with the muscles between the ribs being drawn in with each breath.

▶ Poor circulation: The child looks very pale, and her hands and feet are cold or blue.

▶ Poor feeding: The child has no appetite, and drinks much less than usual. This is especially relevant for infants.

▶ Poor urine output: Again this is especially relevant for infants, where it is noticed that there are fewer wet nappies than usual.

These clinical features cannot be relied on to say for certain that a child is seriously ill, nor does their absence rule out serious illness. If there is any doubt, then medical advice must be sought without delay. The more of the features described above are seen in a child, the more likely it is that she may have a serious illness. Remember that in infants and young children, illness can progress very quickly. If there is any doubt, seek medical advice.

Sudden Infant Death Syndrome (SIDS)

This is the name given to unexpected death in an infant. It happens mostly between one and six months, and is rare after the age of 12 months. The incidence has fallen dramatically in recent years, and the rate is now about 1 in 2000.

Cause

The cause of SIDS is not known, and it is likely due to a number of different causes. Research has focused on immaturity of the infant's breathing, or a defect in the regulation of breathing, or viral infections. It is more common in the winter months and in colder climates (providing a possible link with the baby overheating), and in families from lower socioeconomic groups.

Signs and symptoms

There are no specific features that either predict the event or explain why it happened. In about half the cases parents report a cold or virus infection for a few days before the event, but usually it is so mild that they have not even sought medical advice for it. The child is put down to sleep, and is found dead.

Impact of SIDS

SIDS has a devastating impact on everybody — parents, extended family, siblings, and the professionals involved with the family. Parents will have enormous feelings of guilt, and will play back in minute detail the hours and days leading up to the event, wondering if they missed something, or if they could have done things differently, or if perhaps something they did or did not do may have actually caused or contributed to the death. The grieving process is difficult and prolonged, and in a sense never finishes.

Prevention

Although the cause of SIDS is not known, research has demonstrated associations between a number of factors and SIDS. The reduction of SIDS rates in recent years has been due to the very successful public education campaign designed to make the public aware of these factors.

▶ Sleeping position: Put the baby to sleep on her back or side, with the lower arm well forward so she does not roll over onto her stomach during sleep. There is strong evidence that sleeping on her stomach is a major risk factor for SIDS.

▶ Smoke-free environment: Smoking is associated with an increased risk of SIDS.

▶ Don't overheat the baby: Do not use bumpers in the cot, do not cover her head with a bonnet, do not cover her with too many blankets, and do not overheat the room where she is sleeping.

Implications for early childhood professionals

In the early childhood setting, make sure that the recommendations above are implemented. Although most cases of SIDS occur in the home, some do happen in an early childhood setting. This is a tragedy for all concerned, and is very traumatic for staff. There are a number of support agencies and services available — these can be accessed through the GP, community nurse, children's hospital, or grief and SIDS organisations that can be located in the phone book.

Parents who have experienced SIDS will understandably be anxious about other children, and may be perceived as being overprotective. Early childhood professionals need to be understanding of this situation. If they believe that it is affecting other children in a significant way, they should share this in a sensitive way with the parents and gently suggest to them that they might seek professional help.

Fever

The normal body temperature is about 37° Celsius (98.4°F). It varies during the day, being at its lowest in the morning and a little higher in the late afternoon and evening. Fever is not an illness in itself, but rather the sign of an illness, usually an infection. While sometimes a fever can be present by itself, without anything else to point to the child not being perfectly well, usually there is a runny nose, cough, irritability, poor feeding, vomiting, diarrhoea, and other signs of an infection. The fever is a sign that the body is fighting the infection. The child's temperature will return to normal when the infection has gone. However, in the meantime, it can make the child uncomfortable.

Although the fever may make the child irritable and uncomfortable, the fever itself is not a cause for concern. Many parents worry about a high fever — this has been called 'fever phobia'. While sometimes a high fever may be an important sign of a serious infection, mostly a high fever does not necessarily mean that the child has a serious illness. Most children handle fever well. They may feel cold and shivery when the temperature is rising, and may become mildly dehydrated if the fluid intake is not enough to replace the increased loss due to the fever, or because they do not feel like drinking. Very occasionally a febrile convulsion may be associated with a fever; although this can be frightening for parents they rarely have any long-term consequences. The young child's behaviour is more important than the degree of fever in deciding whether the child may have a serious illness that needs treatment. If the child is alert, playful, socialising normally, eating and drinking well, then it is unlikely that there is any major cause for concern even in the presence of a fever.

The only way to know whether or not the child has a fever is to measure the temperature with a thermometer. Feeling a child's skin (for example by putting lips to the forehead or feeling the brow) is not a reliable way of determining whether fever is present. Plastic tape thermometers placed on the forehead are also not reliable. Children under three usually have their temperature taken by a rectal thermometer (though this is not practical for most early childhood settings), and those over about the age of three are usually cooperative enough to use an oral thermometer (which is put in the mouth for 2 minutes). A better option is to use a digital thermometer that comes with a washable plastic earpiece — the earpiece is inserted gently into the child's ear and produces an accurate recording in seconds. Although fairly expensive, many settings prefer them for their ease of use and the rapidity with which the child's temperature can be ascertained.

Causes of fever

Infections are the commonest cause of a fever in children. Most of these are caused by viruses, which are responsible for upper respiratory infections or colds, some ear infections, and the common childhood illnesses of measles and chickenpox. These infections get better by themselves, and usually no specific treatment is needed.

Other infections are caused by bacteria, and need to be treated with antibiotics. These include some ear infections, tonsillitis, pneumonia, and infections of the urine and blood.

Treatment

Fever is only treated if it is making the child uncomfortable and irritable. A mild fever (less that 38.5°Celsius), if the child looks well, does not need any specific treatment. Here are some general suggestions for what to do when the child has a fever.

▶ Dress the child in light clothing. Even though she may complain of feeling cold, this is because of the fever.

▶ Offer the child extra fluids as the fever increases the amount of fluid that is lost from the body. Water or diluted fruit juices or lemonade are best, unless the child has gastroenteritis (see page 123) in which case oral rehydration fluid is recommended. Most children do better with small amounts of fluid offered more frequently.

▶ Do not worry if the child is not very hungry — this is common when the child has a fever or an infection. Try small amounts of food more often and avoid fatty heavy food, which is more difficult to digest.

▶ Unless the child has other symptoms, there is no reason for her not to go to child care or attend preschool.

▶ There is no reason for a child with a fever to be confined to bed or to rest all the time. Children are very good at determining their own levels of activity when they are sick. Let the child dictate how active she wants to be. Sometimes she will want to lie around, at other times she will want to play.

▶ Cooling measures such as fans, cool baths, and tepid sponging have not been shown to be effective in reducing the fever, and generally are not recommended.

▶ The most effective way to bring the fever down is to use medication. The safest and most widely used is paracetamol (eg Panadol, Tempra, Dymadon). This can be given every 3–4 hours in the correct dose (15 mg of paracetamol for each kg of the child's body weight; it is best to follow the instructions on the bottle or packet unless the doctor recommends a different dose). Paracetamol can also be given as a suppository for those children who are vomiting and have difficulty taking things by mouth.

Aspirin is also very effective in rapidly reducing a fever, but should not be given to infants or young children because of its side effects. It can cause stomach upset, intestinal bleeding and is associated with a rare but potentially fatal condition called Reye Syndrome. Paracetamol is the preferred medicine to treat fever in childhood; aspirin is to be avoided.

When to seek medical advice

Infants under the age of 6 months should always be seen by a doctor. In older children the fever itself is not a concern; in general the child's behaviour is a better indicator of the severity of the illness than the degree of the fever. Seek medical attention if the child does not look well, or looks sicker than previously; if she has difficulty breathing; if she refuses to drink or has persistent vomiting; or becomes drowsy. If the child seems well and happy, even if a little irritable and not eating quite as much, then there is no need to worry about the fever.

If a high fever persists for a couple of days, it is wise to see a doctor to be sure there is nothing serious or no condition that needs treatment.

Prevention

Fever associated with infections are part and parcel of childhood and cannot be prevented.

Conditions of the ear, nose and throat
Colds (upper respiratory tract infections)

Colds are by far the commonest illness in children as well as in adults. The average preschool child has six to eight colds a year, which means that some have considerably more. At times it seems to some parents, especially in the winter months, that the child is constantly sick, barely recovering from one cold before coming down with another. Young children are especially susceptible as their immune systems have not had a chance to build up immunity to the many viruses that are responsible for colds, and their contact with other children at child care or preschool means that they are continually exposed to viruses.

Cause

Colds are caused by one of many viruses; there are believed to be over two hundred different types of viruses that can cause the common cold. Children can contract a cold at any time of the year, though they are more common in the winter months when children are in closer contact with each other as they are indoors and more likely to infect one another. Viruses which cause colds are spread from person to person by sneezing or coughing (droplet spread) or by hand contact — the virus can get onto the fingers after wiping a runny nose.

Signs and symptoms

Children have various combinations of runny or blocked nose, sore throat, cough, headache, swollen and tender glands in the neck, and sometimes fever. They may be irritable and not hungry, and occasionally have nausea and vomiting. There is a great deal of variability in terms of severity and clinical features from one child to another, and from one illness to the next.

The symptoms of a cold are usually not serious, and last for a few days to a week. Very occasionally there are complications such as an ear infection or chest infection.

Treatment

There is no cure for the common cold. There is no specific treatment that will make the cold better more quickly — it just has to run its course. However there are some measures that can help make the child more comfortable.

▶ While she may not feel like eating, lots of fluids are important, and warm drinks may ease a sore throat and dry mouth.

▶ For the older child, lozenges may help ease a sore throat; the cheap ones from the milk bar or supermarket are just as good as expensive ones sold by the chemist.

▶ Nose drops may help if the nose is blocked, though they should not be used for more than a couple of days at a time.

▶ If fever is present and making the child uncomfortable, then paracetamol can be give in appropriate doses (see Fever, page 38).

▶ Let the child decide how active she wants to be; there is no reason to keep the child in bed or to limit her activity, though most children will probably be a little quieter than usual.

▶ There is no reason the child should be excluded from the child care setting if she is otherwise well.

Antibiotics are of no use in the treatment of colds, though they are often prescribed. This is because colds are caused by viruses, against which antibiotics are ineffective. Decongestants, cough medicines and various cold mixtures that can be purchased without a prescription are also often given, but none of these groups of medication has ever been shown to make any difference to the course of the illness, and should not be given to young children.

When to seek medical advice

Colds will almost all get better in a few days without any specific treatment, and mostly visits to the doctor are not necessary. However, if the child has a high and persistent fever, complains of earache or headache, refuses fluids or is vomiting, has difficulty breathing, or does not show signs of improvement after a few days, then a medical consultation is warranted.

Prevention

It is virtually impossible to prevent children from getting upper respiratory tract infections. Giving vitamin C and other vitamins makes no difference, nor does the 'flu injection, which is reserved for children with specific chronic medical conditions.

Tonsillitis

This is part of the spectrum of upper respiratory tract infections, and refers specifically to infection of the tonsils. A child can have tonsillitis alone, though more commonly it is associated with an upper respiratory infection.

Cause

Most commonly tonsillitis is caused by one of many viruses, though sometimes it can be caused by germs (bacteria) such as streptococcus. It can be difficult clinically to tell the difference between a viral and bacterial tonsillitis, so often antibiotics are prescribed.

Signs and symptoms

The child will complain of a sore throat and difficult and painful swallowing. In severe cases this may lead to a reluctance to eat or drink. Often there will be a fever and the glands in the neck will be swollen and tender. There may be associated symptoms such as headache, a blocked or runny nose, and often the child will be quiet or else irritable.

Treatment

Because of the difficulty in differentiating a strep throat from a viral tonsillitis, antibiotics are often prescribed. This is taken as a mixture, capsules or tablets, depending on the age of the child. General treatment is similar to that for a cold — warm drinks, lozenges, and paracetamol for fever. There is no specific need to stay in bed or to rest, though the child may not feel like taking part in many activities, especially in the early stages of the illness. Let the child decide how active she wants to be.

When to seek medical advice

If the throat is painful to the extent that the child has difficulty swallowing, or if the fever is very high, or if there are associated symptoms such as severe headache or drowsiness, or if she does not improve after a few days, then medical assessment is advised.

Prevention

There are no ways in which tonsillitis can be prevented.

Pharyngitis

The signs and symptoms of pharyngitis are very similar to tonsillitis, except it is the back of the throat (the pharynx) rather than the tonsils which are infected. Usually it is caused by a virus, though again antibiotics are often prescribed. The treatment and other features are virtually the same as for tonsillitis.

Influenza

Although people often say they have the 'flu, what they usually have is a cold caused by one of many viruses.

Cause

Influenza is caused by the influenza virus, and is much less common than the usual upper respiratory infections. Influenza tends to occur in winter epidemics.

Signs and symptoms

The symptoms are similar to those seen in upper respiratory tract infections — blocked or runny nose, cough, fever — except there may be more general body symptoms such as aches and pains and headache.

Treatment

Treatment is supportive only, as for a cold. There is no specific treatment for influenza.

When to seek medical advice

Same as for colds (see page 41).

Prevention

There is no effective way to prevent the 'flu. Immunisation is not totally effective, and in any case is not indicated for most children.

Ear infections (otitis media)

Ear infections are one of the commonest infections seen in toddlers and preschool children. Like colds and upper respiratory infections, they occur especially in the winter months. The majority of children will have an occasional ear infection, which will resolve quickly, and mostly ear infections are not serious. Some have recurrent ear infections, and a number of these will develop chronic otitis media or 'glue ear', which can lead to hearing loss (see pages 136–9). This is the main complication of ear infections and if the hearing loss is prolonged or even intermittent, a child's language and communication skills may be affected resulting in delayed language acquisition.

Cause

Ear infections can be caused by bacteria or by viruses; often they are associated with a viral upper respiratory tract infection.

Signs and symptoms

While sometimes ear infections are 'silent' and do not cause any specific symptoms, mostly they are associated with a fever and often an upper respiratory tract infection. General signs of infection may be present, including fever and flushed face, runny nose, loss of appetite, and general misery. There is usually pain in the ear, and infants will cry and may pull at their ear. Some children will have temporary loss of hearing. Occasionally the eardrum may rupture and result in a discharging ear with blood sometimes mixed in. This actually relieves the pain, and makes the child feel better.

Glue ear may not cause any noticeable symptoms at all, or parents or professionals may notice the child does not seem to listen, wants to have things repeated, speaks loudly, or turns the television up loud — all signs of a hearing loss. If a child's language is delayed then hearing loss possibly due to glue ear should be suspected.

Treatment

It is very difficult to know if the cause of the infection is bacterial (where antibiotics are effective) or viral (where antibiotics do not work). For this reason, most children are treated with antibiotics. Paracetamol can help with fever and pain, as can nose drops in some children if they are very blocked up. Blowing the nose is helpful in reducing the pressure felt in the ears, but younger children find this difficult. There is no reason to exclude the child with an ear infection from child care or preschool.

The treatment of glue ear is not straightforward. Some children will be prescribed antibiotics to be taken over a long period, sometimes months.

Others may have surgery to drain their ears and sometimes ventilating tubes (grommets) are inserted.

When to seek medical advice

If the child complains of pain in the ear, or an infant is crying and flushed and pulling at his ear, and especially if a fever is present, or if there is a discharge from the ear, then he should be seen by a doctor. Sometimes the doctor will want to check the child when he is better to make sure the infection has cleared up and there is no evidence of glue ear.

Prevention

Ear infections cannot be prevented, though those that are caused by Haemophilus will not occur if the child is fully immunised. If a child has recurrent ear infections, he should be promptly treated and closely monitored to ensure he does not develop glue ear and subsequent hearing loss.

Swollen glands

Many children will have swollen and sometimes painful glands, most often in their neck. These are lymph glands and are part of the body's defence against infection. These are especially common in the winter months when young children suffer from frequent viral infections. Sometimes the glands are painful, often not, and they can readily be seen at the side of the neck. There is no need to treat swollen glands, and they will slowly reduce in size over time. Rarely, an infected gland will need to be treated with antibiotics and even drained.

Croup

Croup is an infection of the voice box (larynx) which occurs mostly in young children under three years of age. The inflammation causes swelling and the production of mucus which causes the windpipe (trachea) to become narrower and this causes the noisy breathing and croupy cough which is the hallmark of the condition. It is usually associated with a cold or upper respiratory tract infection and is therefore more common in the winter months. Usually the condition is benign and gets better by itself, though occasionally the obstruction to the airway can be severe enough to seriously interfere with the child's breathing so that urgent medical attention and sometimes hospitalisation is required.

Cause

Croup is caused by one of the virus infections that causes the common cold.

Signs and symptoms

The child almost always has symptoms of a cold first — sore throat, irritability, runny nose and fever. He then develops a harsh cough, hoarse voice and noisy breathing which is worse at night and when he is distressed. The noise on breathing is heard as the child breathes in, in contrast to asthma when the noise is heard as the child breathes out. Any activity that increases the rate or force of breathing, such as crying, will make the child sound worse. When the child is quiet or asleep, the noise is quieter and sometimes can hardly be heard.

Most children will get better over a few days; a few will have more severe croup so they will have trouble eating and drinking as well as breathing; these children often end up in hospital for observation and treatment.

Treatment

Most children with croup do not need any treatment and will get better over a few days. Antibiotics are not prescribed because croup is caused by a virus. Steam seems to help some children, though these days it is used less than formerly because there is no really strong evidence that it makes any difference to most children. Nursing the child quietly in a warm room so that he does not get agitated is just as effective and much less trouble. Recent research suggests that a single dose of steroids (prednisolone) taken by mouth is an effective treatment. A child with croup can attend child care or preschool if well enough to take part in the usual activities and if he seems to be over the worst of it.

Croup

When to seek medical advice

The child needs to be seen by a doctor if he is having difficulty with breathing, or if his breathing is noisy at rest.

Prevention

Croup cannot be prevented.

Hay fever/allergic rhinitis

Children suffer hay fever and allergic rhinitis in the same way as adults, with the same range of symptoms.

Cause

The cause is allergies to various substances in the air, often to pollens and grasses, but to a range of other inhaled substances as well. Symptoms are usually worse in spring. There is often a family history of allergy, hay fever, eczema or asthma.

Signs and symptoms

The child will have a blocked or runny nose, which he is often wiping with the back of his hand (the 'allergic salute'). His throat may be dry and sore, his eyes watery and bloodshot, and his ears itchy and blocked.

Treatment

There is no cure, and treatment is directed towards the symptoms. It can include antihistamines to be taken by mouth and steroid nasal sprays. Although a course of desensitisation injections is sometimes advocated, generally there is little evidence of their effectiveness.

Chest and lungs

Asthma

One in five Australian children has asthma, making it the most common chronic medical condition of childhood. Apart from the normal coughs and colds of childhood, it is *the condition most likely to be encountered in early childhood settings*. Not all of these children will have symptoms all of the time. There is a range of severity of asthma, from those children who have only one or two attacks in their lifetime through to those who need to take medications every day. Most children with asthma are able to lead essentially normal lives, provided they receive the correct medical management. It is important that professionals as well as parents have a good understanding of asthma and how it is treated.

Cause

Children with asthma often have other family members who suffer from asthma, hay fever or allergies — there seems to be a genetic predisposition to asthma. Not all children with such a predisposition will go on to develop asthma. There appears to be a trigger early in life which switches on the disease. This can be a viral infection, an allergy of some kind, or an irritant such as cigarette smoke.

In asthma, the smaller airways in the lungs become narrower due to inflammation and then swelling of their walls; in addition there is a lot of mucus production and tightening and spasm of the smooth muscle in the walls. This results in further narrowing of the airways, which reduces the flow of air in and out of the lungs, and is also responsible for the wheeze, cough, and difficulty in breathing that are the hallmarks of acute asthma.

Once a child has asthma, a number of things can trigger an acute attack. The most common trigger is a viral infection. This starts in the usual way with a runny nose, sore throat, slight cough, perhaps a mild fever. In children without asthma this generally runs its course without any specific treatment and gets better over a few days. Children with asthma have hyper-reactive airways, so the viral infection may lead to increasing cough, wheeze, and difficulty breathing.

Other common triggers include exercise and exertion, inhaling cold air, air pollutants such as cigarette smoke or paint fumes, and allergens such as animal hair, especially cats.

Signs and symptoms

The child will have wheeze, cough, tightness in the chest, shortness of breath, and noisy breathing. The exact symptoms will vary according to how severe the attack is.

In very mild cases, wheeze may not be heard unless the doctor listens to the child's chest with a stethoscope. The child may have a cough, especially at night time or after running around, and be just a little off-colour. In more severe cases, the wheeze will be easily heard. The child may also show signs of respiratory distress such as rapid breathing, tugging of the muscles of the neck, and difficulty breathing and may have difficulty speaking more than a few words at a time because of shortness of breath. A severe attack is scary both for the child and for the professionals. Most children with asthma have milder symptoms.

It is sometimes not realised that cough is very much part of asthma. It is commonly thought that because a child does not have a wheeze, then she does not have asthma. However the cough, usually worse at night or after exercise, may affect the child's life almost as much as the wheeze and shortness of breath. The cough in asthma will often sound moist or fruity and older children may bring up yellow or greenish phlegm.

In some children there may be neither a wheeze nor cough, but the child may complain of tightness in the chest, of feeling tired or off-colour, or be less interested in food. The symptoms of asthma can sometimes be vague.

There is great variability in the severity and frequency of children's asthma. A small number of children have chronic persistent asthma and need to take several medications every day. Some have only one or two attacks. Others have what is called episodic asthma — in between attacks they have no or very mild symptoms, but wheeze and cough when they have a cold or viral infection, especially during the winter months or during the spring pollen season.

Treatment

The first principle of treatment is to try to prevent attacks from occurring at all. If acute attacks do occur, or symptoms are present, then the aim is to limit both their severity and duration. For many children, the most effective treatment of asthma is to take medications every day to prevent attacks — these are children who would otherwise have attacks relatively frequently. Most children have only occasional attacks and do not need to take preventive medication — they take medication only when they have symptoms. More children with asthma get into trouble because they are undertreated than because they use medications too much.

Medications used in asthma can be divided into **relievers** and **preventers**.

Relievers are quick acting and are used to treat the symptoms of an attack, so they are given when the child begins to cough and wheeze. They act on the smooth muscle surrounding the breathing tubes to make them wider and so relieve the symptoms. They are usually given by inhalation every three to four hours though, if the symptoms are severe, can be given safely more frequently. These medications include Ventolin, Respolin, Serevent, Bricanyl, Berotec, and Atrovent. Steroids (prednisone) are also often given (by mouth) during an acute attack. Relievers are also used before exercise or sport in those children who get symptoms such as cough, wheeze or shortness of breath when they exert themselves. The child takes a dose of medication just before the activity begins, and again during it if needed.

Preventers are used to prevent attacks or daily symptoms, and include Intal, Becotide, Pulmicort and Flixatide. These are usually given once or twice a day. A minority of children need to take steroid tablets every day to keep their asthma under control. Some children take both preventers and relievers.

Asthma medications are generally given by inhalation. Children from about the age of 7–8 years of age are able to use puffers. Younger children are able to use the puffers in conjunction with a 'spacer', which is a plastic cylinder. The puffer fits into one end and the child then puts her lips over the other end and takes half a dozen deep breaths. Toddlers are able to use these devices which deliver the medication directly into the lungs. Sometimes a nebuliser is used — this is an electrical pump and the medication is turned into a fine mist via an air pump. This is especially useful in an acute attack, though for most children medication delivered by a spacer device is likely to be just as effective.

Treatment of an acute attack

Every child with asthma should have a written asthma action plan so it is clear exactly what needs to be done during an acute attack. This should be obtained from the child's doctor via the parent at the time the child is enrolled.

The general plan should be as follows:

▶ Sit with the child in a quiet place and make sure she stays calm.

▶ Give the reliever medication several times over an hour, and then every 3–4 hours.

▶ If this does not control the symptoms, or if they are getting worse, then seek medical advice as soon as possible, or go to a hospital emergency department.

▶ If the child is very distressed — going blue around the lips or having great difficulty breathing or is unable to talk — call an ambulance and give the child a reliever medication by inhaler or nebuliser every few minutes.

When to seek medical advice

The child should be seen by a doctor if:

▶ the symptoms are troublesome and not responding to the usual medication;

▶ the child needs medicine first thing in the morning or more frequently than usual;

▶ the child gets short of breath when running around and cannot keep up with her peers; and

▶ an acute attack needs medication more often than every 2–3 hours.

Cough

Cough is one of the commonest symptoms in preschool children, especially in the winter months. Sometimes it can linger for weeks and is distressing to the child and her caregivers.

Cause

Cough associated with or persisting after a viral infection is by far the commonest cause of cough. The child may have the cough during the acute phase, and it can persist for a long time after the child is otherwise recovered from the cold. Asthma is also common and needs to be considered, especially if the child is a known asthmatic or if she has wheezed before or has a family history of asthma. Other, less common, causes of cough include exposure to smoke or cold air, which irritates the airways, inhaled foreign body, other viral infections such as croup or bronchiolitis, or whooping cough in a child who is not immunised.

Signs and symptoms

The nature of the cough and its severity vary according to the cause. The cough of asthma is often worse at night and may be associated with a wheeze or shortness of breath. A cough following a cold is also worse at night and on exertion, but the child is otherwise well. Fever, sore throat and irritability suggest an acute infection.

Treatment

Treatment of cough depends on its cause. If it is due to asthma or to an acute viral infection, then these conditions should be treated appropriately as described above. Antibiotics are only prescribed where there is a clear indication, for example a bacterial infection.

However for the commonest cause of persistent cough, that which follows a viral infection, there is no effective treatment. Cough medicines, decongestants, and antihistamines are often used but there is no real evidence that they make any difference to either the intensity or duration of the cough, and they may cause side effects such as drowsiness, irritability and rapid heart rate.

When to seek medical advice

If the cough is severe enough to interfere with the child's day-to-day functioning, or persists for weeks, then she should be seen by a doctor.

Prevention

If the cough is due to asthma, then it is likely that it can be prevented by appropriate medication.

Bronchiolitis

Bronchiolitis is a viral infection of the small air passages of the lungs (bronchioles). It occurs especially in the winter months and is commonest in infants under 12 months of age.

Cause

Bronchiolitis is caused by a virus (respiratory syncytial virus (RSV)), which is spread by sneezing, coughing or personal contact.

Signs and symptoms

The infection begins like a cold, with runny nose and mild cough and perhaps a slight fever. Over the next couple of days the cough becomes worse and the breathing laboured and rapid. Often a wheeze is heard when the infant breathes out. Sometimes the symptoms become so severe that they interfere with the infant's feeding and she can find it hard to breathe and becomes quite distressed. In most cases the infection is mild and the symptoms begin to get better over a few days

Treatment

There is no specific treatment for bronchiolitis. Most infants have a mild infection that can be managed at home; if the condition is severe enough that the baby is distressed with her breathing and it makes feeding difficult, then admission to hospital may be necessary. Fluid intake should be increased, and paracetamol will help reduce the fever and make the infant more comfortable. The young child with bronchiolitis does not need to be excluded from the early childhood setting if it is mild and not getting worse.

When to seek medical advice

If bronchiolitis is suspected — the child is coughing and wheezing and breathing rapidly — then medical assessment is required. The doctor should see the child urgently if the breathing is becoming more laboured, the cough and wheeze getting worse, if there is blueness around the lips, or an infant is having trouble with eating and drinking.

Prevention

Bronchiolitis tends to occur in epidemics in the winter months. Infection is either by droplet spread or personal contact, and spread can be minimised by attention to routine hygiene and infection control practices (see page 10).

Bronchitis

Bronchitis is an infection of the larger breathing tubes (bronchi) of the lungs, and can be caused by viruses and bacteria. It is seen in adults but is very uncommon in children. In the past, children were diagnosed as having 'wheezy bronchitis', but this term is not used now — the condition referred to is likely to be asthma. If bronchitis is suspected, it is likely to be something else and a medical assessment is required to make the correct diagnosis and institute appropriate treatment.

Pneumonia

Pneumonia is an infection of the lungs, and can occur in children at any age. It can cause serious illness and often, especially in younger children, hospitalisation is necessary.

Cause

Pneumonia can be caused by viruses or bacteria or other germs (for example, mycoplasma). Sometimes it can be seen as a complication of another infection (for example, whooping cough) or be associated with an underlying condition such as cystic fibrosis.

Signs and symptoms

These will vary with the age of the child and the type of infection. Infants and younger children are often very sick, with rapid and distressed breathing and cough. In older children there is persistent cough, sometimes chest pain, fever, and rapid and laboured breathing. The diagnosis is made by listening to the chest with a stethoscope and confirmed by a chest X-ray.

Treatment

Infants and young children almost always need hospital treatment, at least initially. Older children with mild illness can be treated at home, though close medical supervision is necessary. Antibiotics are given if it is suspected that the infection may be bacterial. They are continued for a week or longer, or until the child is well again. Sometimes a repeat chest X-ray is performed some weeks later to make sure the infection has cleared up completely.

When to seek medical advice

If pneumonia is suspected — the child looks unwell and has a fever and a persistent and distressing cough — then medical assessment is advised. If pneumonia has already been diagnosed and the child is not getting better after a few days, or seems to be getting worse, then reassessment is advised.

Prevention

Pneumonia cannot really be prevented though, if it is viral, then hygiene and infection control practices can prevent it being spread (see page 10). Contrary to common folklore, pneumonia cannot be contracted by going outside in cold or rainy weather.

Pertussis (whooping cough)

See under Infectious diseases, page 77.

Eyes

Conjunctivitis

Conjunctivitis is an infection or irritation of the lining (conjunctiva) over the eyeball and inside the eyelids. It is common in young children and is very contagious.

Cause

Usually conjunctivitis is caused by an infection with a virus or bacteria, but it can also be due to irritation of the eye due to an object or chemical that has entered the eye, or to an allergic reaction. Sometimes it can occur as part of a cold with the same virus causing both conditions.

Signs and symptoms

The child's eye will be red and teary, and she might complain of sand in the eye or use other words to describe a grittiness in the eye. Sometimes there will be a greenish thick discharge from the eye, and when the child wakes from sleep the eyelids may be puffy and stuck together. The child will be constantly rubbing her eye because of the discomfort, and in this way can easily spread the infection to the other eye. The child may have symptoms of a cold (see page 41).

Treatment

The eye is washed and cleaned gently several times a day with cotton wool soaked in warm water. If the conjunctivitis is associated with a cold, it is most likely to be viral and no other treatment is necessary. Otherwise it is often difficult to tell the difference between a viral and bacterial infection, and eye drops and/or ointment may be prescribed. If the conjunctivitis is due to another cause — irritation due to something in the eye or to allergy — then this is treated according to the cause. The eye may be washed with water to wash away a chemical, or the allergy treated with eye drops. It is best to exclude a child who has conjunctivitis from child care or preschool until there is no more discharge or tearing from the affected eye.

When to seek medical advice

It is best to have a doctor check a child with conjunctivitis, unless it is mild or part of a cold. Medical advice should always be sought if the child is also unwell, or if the conjunctivitis does not clear up after a few days.

Prevention

Conjunctivitis in young children cannot be prevented. However, it is possible to prevent the spread of infection from one child to another with proper hygiene and infection control procedures, for example having the child not use a common towel and other articles and having her wash her hands after rubbing her eyes. (See also Exclusion Table, page 79.)

Vision difficulties requiring glasses

Many children wear glasses because of problems with vision. They need lenses to correct problems with their visual acuity, or in some cases wear glasses as treatment for amblyopia (see below, page 64). Early childhood professionals may be the first to suspect that a child has problems with vision. They may notice that the child peers very closely at objects, or holds a book very close to his eyes, or seems not very interested in visual or visual-motor activities. If a vision problem is suspected as a result of these or other observations, the early childhood professional should share these observations with parents and suggest that the child's eyes be checked by a specialist, preferably by an ophthalmologist (medically trained eye specialist) who is experienced in working with young children.

Short-sightedness (myopia)

Children who have myopia can see things close up but have difficulty seeing distant objects clearly. It is the most common visual acuity problem in young children, and is due to an eyeball that is longer than average. It tends to run in families, and usually gets worse as children approach adolescence. Children with myopia sit very close to the television, hold a book close to their eyes, and in class may have difficulty seeing the blackboard clearly. The treatment is to wear corrective lenses; in young children this invariably means glasses rather than contact lenses. The lenses of the glasses need to be checked every six months or so to make sure they are correct for the growing eye.

Long-sightedness (hyperopia)

This is a condition in which the eyeball is shorter than average, making it difficult for the child to see things up close. Most children are long-sighted at birth but as the eye grows the condition corrects itself, and glasses are not usually needed unless it is severe. If glasses are needed it is only for close-up work, and the child does not need to wear them all of the time. Because the child is straining to see things close up, activities such as reading may cause fatigue, eye discomfort, and sometimes headaches.

Astigmatism

Astigmatism is an uneven curvature of the surface of the eyeball (lens and cornea). This may cause vision to be blurred. It is treated with corrective lenses, so the child needs to wear glasses.

Squint (strabismus, crossed eyes)

Squint is sometimes evident from birth, or else becomes noticeable at a few months of age. It is an important condition to detect, for if it is not corrected it may lead to amblyopia (see below, page 64).

Cause

Squint is usually due to an imbalance of the muscles of the eyes. Each eye has a series of muscles which make the eyes move in synchrony with each other. If one of the muscles is weak, then that eye does not move in synchrony with the other and results in the squint. Very rarely the squint is caused by something else, such as a tumour in the eye or an abnormality of another part of the eye.

Signs and symptoms

While it is not uncommon for a newborn baby's eyes to wander, within a few weeks he learns to move his eyes together, and any persistence after this means the child has a squint. Usually one eye is affected, and may turn inwards, outwards, or wander. The result is that the eyes of a child with squint appear to be looking in different directions. Sometimes this is obvious all the time, and in other children it becomes more pronounced when they are tired. Some children have a facial appearance that makes them appear that they have a squint, although their eyes are perfectly aligned. This is because they have prominent folds alongside the nose (epicanthic folds).

Treatment

It is critically important that the child's eyes are perfectly aligned in order that they move in synchrony with each other, so it is important that the child is seen by an ophthalmologist as soon as the squint is diagnosed so a treatment plan can be devised. The treatment varies according to the severity and cause, but may involve a combination of drops, glasses, patching and surgery. Children do not grow out of a squint, and active treatment is always necessary.

When to seek medical advice

As soon as the squint is evident, no matter how young the child, he should be seen by a doctor and referred to a paediatrician or ophthalmologist.

Prevention

While squint cannot be prevented, amblyopia, which is a serious complication of squint, can be prevented with early and appropriate treatment.

Amblyopia

Ambylopia is a loss of vision in one eye. A child with ambylopia has functioning vision in only one eye.

Cause

Amblyopia can result from injury or disease in one eye, from a major refractive error in one eye, or most commonly as a complication of squint. If one eye does not see well as a result of injury or refractive error, the 'good eye' begins to be used more, and the weak or 'lazy' eye becomes less active and even weaker. If there is a squint, and the eyes are not perfectly aligned, the child may have double vision because the images coming from the eyes to the brain are different. The brain then suppresses the image from the 'lazy' eye to get rid of the double vision, and the vision in the affected eye is reduced further.

Signs and symptoms

Amblyopia is very difficult to detect without a formal vision test. Sometimes it may be noticed that the child turns his head to one side when looking at things.

Treatment

This depends on the cause. If it is due to refractive error, then corrective lenses in the form of glasses will usually be all that is needed. Sometimes the child wears a patch over the good eye in order to force him to use and strengthen the eye that has become 'lazy'. Alternatively, sometimes glasses with an opaque lens over the good eye are prescribed, or sometimes eye drops to blur the vision in the good eye. Treatment will begin as soon as the condition is diagnosed and may last months or even years.

Treatment of amblyopia has implications for child care staff and teachers, and they must be certain to obtain detailed information from the parents and the treating doctor about what is expected from them in the out-of-home situation.

When to seek medical advice

If there is any concern about a child's vision or appearance of his eyes at any age, then medical assessment by a specialist is very important.

Prevention

Amblyopia due to squint or refractive errors is preventable with early diagnosis and treatment.

Stye

A stye is a small pimple which forms at the edge of an eyelid around an eyelash.

Cause

The cause is a bacterial infection of the cells surrounding the hair follicles or sweat glands on the edge of the eyelid.

Signs and symptoms

A stye is a red, raised lump which looks just like a pimple on the base of an eyelash. It is uncomfortable and can be quite painful as well as unsightly.

Treatment

A stye will eventually go away without any specific treatment, and will often drain itself. Bathing the affected eye for 10–15 minutes several times a day with cotton wool that has been soaked in warm water will often help speed the process as well as being soothing.

When to seek medical advice

Specific medical treatment is not necessary. Medical advice should be sought if it does not resolve within a few days, if it is very large and causing pain, or if it recurs frequently.

Foreign body in eye

This information is dealt with under 'Emergencies, Foreign bodies' (see page 28).

A word about eyes for early childhood professionals

The information reaching the brain through the visual pathways is essential for normal development. Visual impairment may significantly handicap a child's ability to learn and relate to the outside world. Often early childhood professionals are in a position where they are the first to suspect that a young child has a problem with vision. It is important to try to detect vision problems as early as possible. Often early treatment can make a big difference to the child and to the eventual outcomes.

Some signs of possible eye problems requiring early referral for specialist opinion include:

▶ squint;

▶ holding a book very close or sitting close to the TV or board;

▶ squinting when looking at distant objects such as the blackboard or people a long way away;

▶ screwing up of eyes or squinting when looking at objects up close;

▶ holding books at arms-length, and complaining of blurriness if holding it at normal distance; and

▶ complaints of headache or sore eyes after working up close, for example looking at a book.

Children take to wearing glasses with differing degrees of acceptance, depending on their age and temperament. The younger the child usually the more problematic it may be. Glasses can be made with unbreakable lenses and frames, so breakage is not usually a problem. Forgetting to wear them often is, and the professional may need to remind and encourage the child to wear them. Some children with glasses are teased, and this needs to be handled quickly and firmly.

Often more problematic is the child undergoing treatment for amblyopia whose eye needs to be patched. While the 'lazy' eye is being strengthened by forcing the child to use it, vision may be a problem, especially early in the course of treatment, and this needs to be taken into account in the way the child is handled and taught. They will usually need closer supervision, especially in the playground where their depth perception is likely to be inaccurate so they may be prone to accidents.

Infectious diseases
Chickenpox (varicella)

Chickenpox is one of the commonest infectious diseases of childhood, though it can also occur in adults where it is not as mild as in young children.

Cause

Chickenpox is caused by the varicella virus. It is highly contagious, being spread by droplet infection (coughing and sneezing), direct contact with contaminated objects, or direct contact from person to person, and has an incubation period of 10 to 21 days. The infectious period lasts from a few days before the rash appears until all the existing lesions are dried up and no longer weeping, which takes about a week from the onset of the rash.

Signs and symptoms

The illness begins with non-specific signs of illness such as tiredness, lethargy, and mild fever, and is followed a few days later by the first appearance of the distinctive rash which is the hallmark of chickenpox. The rash looks like small red spots which quickly turn into blisters with white tops filled with a clear fluid that burst easily and form scabs or crusts. They appear in crops initially over the body and scalp, and then arms, legs, and sometimes the mouth, ears and genitalia. New crops keep on appearing each day as the older spots begin to scab and dry up. The rash is extremely itchy, and occasionally it becomes infected because of the child's scratching.

In healthy children, complications of chickenpox — pneumonia and encephalitis (inflammation of the lining of the brain) — are rare, except for scarring and secondary infection due to scratching. In childhood the illness is usually relatively mild, with some fever and constitutional upset, but the child is rarely very sick. The itchiness of the rash causes the most distress. New crops of spots keep on appearing for about a week and then stop, though it may take some time for them all to dry up completely and disappear.

Treatment

There is no specific treatment for chickenpox and the illness runs an uneventful and predictable course. Treatment is geared to relieving the symptoms. Calamine lotion is soothing and can be helpful. The child's nails should be cut short to lessen the chances of scarring and secondary infection, or in younger children mittens can be used, especially at night time. The child should not attend day care or preschool until the rash is scabbed over and completely dry and no new lesions are occurring.

When to seek medical advice

Apart from the initial consultation where the diagnosis is made, there is usually no need to seek further medical advice unless there are complications or the child appears sick.

Prevention

Because chickenpox is highly contagious, the spread maybe decreased by attention to the usual hygiene and infection control procedures (see page 10). Once the child has had chickenpox she is immune and will not get it again, though the virus lies dormant and may cause shingles in adult life. A chickenpox vaccine is now available. At the time of writing, it was recommended as part of the immunisation schedule but not funded, so parents have to make arrangements with the child's GP to administer it. (See also Exclusion Table, page 79.)

Glandular fever

Glandular fever is a common viral illness which affects mainly older children and adolescents, but glandular fever type illnesses can be seen also in younger children.

Cause

Glandular fever is caused by a virus called the Epstein-Barr virus, and is commonly transmitted through saliva (hence its nickname in adolescents as 'the kissing disease'). However there are a number of other viruses that cause symptoms and signs that are almost identical to glandular fever.

Signs and symptoms

The child will have a sore throat and fever, and the glands in the neck are swollen and tender. A red, spotty rash may appear on the trunk — this is flat and fades after a few days. The illness is accompanied by tiredness and lethargy, and a marked loss of appetite. The diagnosis is made by a blood test.

Treatment

Because this is a viral illness, there is no specific treatment or cure. Treatment is directed towards relieving symptoms, such as giving paracetamol if the child is uncomfortable because of the fever, and making sure that he drinks sufficient quantities of fluids.

When to seek medical advice

A doctor will likely be the one who makes the initial diagnosis, and will need to be consulted again if there is no improvement in symptoms after 3–4 days, though this is an illness that can sometimes drag on for weeks.

Hand, foot and mouth disease

This is a common condition in young children, so called because of the location of the blisters which are characteristic of the condition. It is very contagious and spreads easily from one child to the next.

Cause

The condition is caused by a specific virus called Coxsackie A.

Signs and symptoms

The incubation period is about 4–6 days. The child may have a slight fever and be off-colour and without an appetite for a day or two before the rash appears. Small ulcers appear in the child's mouth causing pain and discomfort, and then small blisters appear on the hands and feet, especially on the palms and the soles. The rash clears up after about a week.

Treatment

There is no specific treatment for this condition. The child needs to be encouraged to drink to avoid dehydration, though this may be a problem because of the ulcers present in the mouth. Giving small drinks at frequent intervals is often the key, and icy poles or ice blocks may sometimes be easier because of their coldness which 'freezes' the inside of the mouth and makes the discomfort less. Paracetamol may lessen the pain and lower the fever if it is high.

Hand, foot and mouth disease is a minor illness in young children; it generally runs its course and clears up quickly without any problems.

When to seek medical advice

If the child is refusing to drink or looks sick then medical advice should be sought.

Prevention

Hand, foot and mouth disease is highly infectious and spread mainly by direct contact. The likelihood of spread may be reduced by the usual hygiene and infection control measures (see page 10). (See Exclusion Table, page 79.)

Measles

Measles is a highly contagious and potentially serious disease, seen less commonly these days because of the success of immunisation, but outbreaks still occur from time to time in children who are not immunised. It is a particularly serious disease in malnourished children in developing countries.

Cause

Measles is caused by a virus and is spread rapidly by airborne droplets (coughing and sneezing) or else by direct contact with secretions from the nose or mouth. There is an incubation period of 8–10 days.

Signs and symptoms

Initially the illness is very much like the common cold — runny nose, fever, sore red eyes and a dry hacking cough. The child will be listless and irritable and off her food. The child's mouth may become sore, and small white spots appear inside the cheeks, which are called 'Koplik's spots'. The typical rash of measles appears on the third or fourth day of the illness. It consists of numerous small red patches which begin behind the ears and along the hairline and spread quickly to the rest of the face, and then to the rest of the body. The patches join together and become blotchy, and later the skin may peel a little as the rash fades after 3–5 days. When the rash appears the fever usually increases, and the child feels unwell and miserable.

Very occasionally, but more commonly in some other countries and communities, measles can cause complications such as otitis media, pneumonia, and encephalitis (inflammation of the lining of the brain).

Treatment

There is no specific treatment for measles. Paracetamol is given for the fever, especially after the rash appears when the temperature is usually very high. The child is encouraged to drink fluids, and will not feel much like running around, though bed rest is not essential. She may complain of sore eyes and that the bright light makes it worse, so dimming the lights or keeping the room darkened maybe be helpful. The child should be kept at home to minimise the risk of spread to other children.

When to seek medical advice

Medical consultation should be sought when the rash appears, to confirm that it is measles. Often parents will seek advice before the rash appears because the child is sick and miserable. The presence of fever, cough, red eyes and Koplik's spots will herald the disease even before the rash appears. If there is earache or persistent cough, then the child should be reviewed to make sure that no complications such as otitis media or pneumonia have developed.

Prevention

Measles immunisation (as part of the MMR (measles, mumps and rubella) that is given at 12 months of age and again at 4 years — see Immunisation, page 11) protects the vast majority of children from measles. The child is infectious a few days before the rash appears, so preventing the infection from spreading is difficult. Making sure that all children are fully immunised is the best way of preventing the spread of measles. (See also Exclusion Table, page 79.)

Meningococcal disease

This is a severe and sometimes dramatic infection that causes a number of deaths in Australia each year, both in children (especially under the age of 5 years) and adults (especially late teens and young adults). Despite the publicity that follows an outbreak of infection or a death from meningococcal disease, it is still a rare disease in Australia.

Cause

Meningococcal disease is caused by Neisseria meningitidis, a germ that can be found living harmlessly in the back of the throat of many people. It is when it invades the brain and causes blood poisoning, or infects the lining of the brain and causes meningitis, that it causes problems. The disease does not occur in those who carry the germ, but rather in those who have recently acquired the germ from a healthy carrier. It is spread by droplet contact or from saliva, for example by kissing or sharing utensils or cups that have been used by an infected person. It is more common in winter and early spring.

Signs and symptoms

The disease begins in a similar way to influenza and other viral infections — fever, aches and pains in the muscles, and sometimes vomiting. Some develop the clinical features of meningitis — severe headache, stiff neck, and an intolerance to light. Most will develop the rash which is characteristic of meningococcal disease; these are small red/purple spots which can appear anywhere on the body, but then often and rapidly join up and become a dark purple in colour. The rash does not fade when pressure is applied to it. The condition can progress extremely quickly and the child or adult who was seemingly well can be gravely ill within the space of hours. It is this dramatic nature of the course of the illness, and its potential seriousness, that understandably makes parents and professionals anxious and captures the attention of the media.

Treatment

The meningococcal germ is very sensitive to penicillin, and a few doses of penicillin given early in the course of the disease almost always completely eradicates the bacteria from the bloodstream. The problem is that often the disease is well established by the time it is diagnosed and treatment commenced. All children with meningococcal disease are admitted to hospital.

Household contacts and others who have had close contact with the infected child in the week prior to the onset of the illness — including other children and staff at the early childhood setting — are usually given antibiotics and closely monitored to ensure that they do not become sick.

When to seek medical advice

Any child who has symptoms suggestive of meningitis, or is unwell with a fever and rash, should be seen by a doctor as soon as possible.

Prevention

There are two main subtypes of meningococcus that cause serious disease — types B and C. These each cause about half the cases in Australia each year. While there is no vaccine against type B (as yet), there recently has become available an effective vaccine against type C. This was added in 2003 to the standard immunisation schedule and children aged 1–5 years are now also eligible to receive the vaccine.

The implementation of basic hygiene measures will also reduce the chances of spread of the disease — covering mouth when coughing or sneezing, washing hands, and not sharing cups and utensils that may have saliva on them. (See Exclusion Table, page 79.)

Mumps

Mumps causes inflammation and swelling of the salivary glands beneath the jaw. It is very uncommon these days because of the success of immunisation.

Cause

Mumps is caused by a virus. The incubation period is 2–3 weeks. It is spread by droplet infection (coughing or sneezing) or by contact with infected materials.

Signs and symptoms

The illness begins with a few days of vague, non-specific symptoms such as mild fever and just not feeling well. The child then develops soreness and swelling in the neck in the region of the salivary glands, especially in the parotid gland which is in the angle of the jaw just below the ear. Usually the swelling is confined to one side of the face, although it can be present on both sides. The swollen glands are very tender to touch, and because chewing is painful the child may not feel like eating. In addition to the swollen salivary glands, there can also be abdominal pain, inflammation, swelling and pain in the joints and in the testes in boys.

Treatment

There is no specific treatment for mumps. The child should be made as comfortable as possible with rest, fluids and paracetamol for fever. Chewing solid foods may be painful so food is given in liquid form whenever possible.

When to seek medical advice

If it is suspected that the child may have mumps, a doctor should be consulted to confirm the diagnosis. There are other causes of swollen and painful glands in the neck, and it is important that the correct diagnosis is made.

Prevention

Mumps can be prevented by mumps immunisation, part of the combined MMR (mumps, measles and rubella) that is given routinely at 12 months of age and again at 4 years. (See Exclusion Table, page 79.)

Rubella (German measles)

Rubella in children is a very mild illness which sometimes even passes unnoticed. Its significance lies in the fact that if a pregnant woman acquires rubella in the first three months of pregnancy it can lead to very serious and life threatening congenital defects in the baby. These can include blindness, deafness, mental retardation and heart abnormalities.

Cause

Rubella is caused by a virus which is spread through personal contact or droplets in the air due to coughing and sneezing. The incubation period is 2–3 weeks.

Signs and symptoms

The onset of rubella is rather like a mild cold, with a slight fever, sore throat and enlarged lymph glands in the neck. The characteristic rash appears 2–3 days later. It begins on the face, and spreads to the trunk. The spots are at first a pale pink in colour, and soon merge to form patches. The rash lasts only a few days and then disappears. During this time the child remains mildly unwell with swollen glands in the neck and back of the head.

Treatment

There is no specific treatment. The child is kept comfortable with fluids, rest if needed and paracetamol for the fever.

When to seek medical advice

The main reason to see a doctor is to establish the diagnosis so that the affected child can be kept away from pregnant women. Because of the success of immunisation, rubella is much less common these days, and women who are not immune are advised to have rubella immunisation at least three months before trying to get pregnant.

Prevention

Rubella can be prevented by immunisation; MMR (measles, mumps and rubella) is given routinely at 12 months and again at 4 years. (See Exclusion Table, page 79.)

Whooping cough (pertussis)

Whooping cough is a highly contagious infection of the respiratory tract. It is a very serious and potentially fatal condition, especially in infants and young children. It occurs often in epidemics, especially in young children who are not immunised. A child with whooping cough should not attend child care or preschool.

Cause

Whooping cough is caused by a bacteria which invades the lining of the breathing tubes of the lungs and produces thick mucus. This causes the distressing cough which is characteristic of this condition. It is most commonly spread by droplet infection — coughing and sneezing — and by personal contact. A child can remain infectious for several weeks after the onset of the cough.

Signs and symptoms

The incubation period is one to two weeks. The illness begins much like a cold, with runny nose, watery eyes, sneezing and a mild fever. The cough is mild at first, often at night, and worsens gradually and soon takes on the characteristic features of the condition. The child coughs several times in a row without being able to take a breath in between, and then gasps for a deep breath. The whoop often accompanies the pulling in of air at the end of the coughing fit. The child's face will turn red and often he will vomit in association with the coughing, and may turn blue for a moment until he can breathe in enough air. The whole episode is exhausting for the child, and it interferes with feeding and with sleep. It is distressing for the child and the caregiver alike. In between bouts of coughing, the child may look quite well. This illness can last for weeks before improvement is seen, and some cough may persist for months.

Ear infections (otitis media) and pneumonia are relatively common complications.

Treatment

There is no specific treatment of whooping cough. The child is made comfortable as best one can, and it is important that fluids be taken in sufficient quantities to avoid dehydration. Antibiotics (erythromycin) can reduce the period of infection but do not alter the course of the disease. Children under one year of age are almost always hospitalised.

When to seek medical advice

Medical advice must be sought if whooping cough is suspected. The diagnosis is usually made clinically and confirmed by taking a swab from high up in the child's nose.

Prevention

Early childhood settings are especially vulnerable to epidemics of pertussis, and care should be taken to ensure that every child is fully immunised. (See also Exclusion Table, page 79.)

Exclusion Table

An important part of infection control is to exclude children with certain infections from early childhood settings to ensure that the infection does not spread to other children. The health authorities in each state/territory have published infectious disease regulations which set out the minimum period of exclusion of children and their contacts. Unfortunately, there are no common national regulations, and there are variations from state to state, although these are generally minor. The ones listed below are adapted from those issued by the Victorian Department of Human Services, and are likely to be very similar to those in other states/territories. However, every early childhood setting should obtain the schedule from their relevant state/territory health authority and comply with them. The ones below should be taken as a guide only.

Chickenpox	Exclude until fully recovered or for at least 5 days after the eruption first appears. Some remaining scabs are not a reason for continued exclusion. Contacts do not need to be excluded.
Conjunctivitis	Exclude until discharge from eye has ceased. Contacts do not need to be excluded.
Diarrhoea	Exclude until diarrhoea has ceased. Contacts do not need to be excluded.
Glandular fever	Exclusion not necessary. Contacts do not need to be excluded.
Hand, foot and mouth disease	Exclude until all blisters have dried. Contacts do not need to be excluded.
Head lice	Exclude until the day following treatment. Contacts do not need to be excluded.
Impetigo	Exclude until treatment has commenced. Sores on exposed surfaces must be covered with a watertight dressing. Contacts do not need to be excluded.
Influenza and influenza type illnesses	Exclude until well. Contacts do not need to be excluded.

Exclusion Table (*continued*)

Measles	Exclude for at least 4 days after onset of rash. Contacts do not need to be excluded unless unimmunised.
Meningitis	Exclude until well. Contacts do not need to be excluded.
Meningococcal disease	Exclude until contacts and carriers have begun preventive treatment. Contacts not excluded provided they have begun preventive treatment.
Mumps	Exclude for 9 days or until swelling goes down (whichever is sooner). Contacts do not need to be excluded.
Pertussis (whooping cough)	Exclude until 5 days after beginning antibiotic treatment. Contacts excluded if unimmunised for 14 days after last exposure or until they have taken 5 days of a 10-day course of antibiotics.
Ringworm	Exclude until the day following commencement of treatment. Contacts do not need to be excluded.
Scabies	Exclude until the day following treatment. Contacts do not need to be excluded.
Rubella	Exclude until fully recovered or for at least 4 days after the onset of the rash. Contacts do not need to be excluded.
Worms	Exclude if diarrhoea is present. Contacts do not need to be excluded.

Infections and early childhood staff

Staff working in early childhood settings will inevitably be exposed to young children with infectious diseases, and they will certainly contract more than their fair share of infections, more so than if they were working in other settings where they did not come into such intense and continued contact with young children.

Most of these infections are not serious and are part and parcel of everyday life, especially in the winter months. They can be minimised by attention to good hygiene and infection control practices (see page 10). All staff should make sure they are fully immunised against the vaccine preventable conditions, some of which are very serious and even life threatening. If they are in any doubt about whether they are covered against these common preventable infections, they should consult their doctor, who can check their immune status with a simple blood test and, if necessary, provide vaccination for them.

This is especially important in the case of rubella for women who may be pregnant, considering pregnancy, or of child bearing age. In most cases they will have been vaccinated in childhood with the rubella vaccine as part of the regular immunisation schedule. However if they are uncertain, the safest thing is to have their immune status checked by their doctor. A blood test will determine if they are protected or not. If they are susceptible to infection, then they should have the rubella vaccine before beginning work in an early childhood setting.

Skin

Birthmarks

Various marks or blemishes are often present on a baby's skin from birth. Most will fade with time, though some persist.

Salmon patches ('stork bites')

These are pale pink marks which are seen on the baby's forehead, eyelids, bridge of nose, and/or the back of the head and neck. They are called stork marks because they correspond to where the beak of the stork would hold the infant as it brings it into the world. Salmon patches slowly lighten and fade and have largely disappeared by the toddler stage.

Strawberry haemangioma

These are dilated blood vessels just under the skin. They are usually small and sometimes hardly noticeable at birth, but over the next six months or so they grow quickly in size and become raised, reddish/purple in colour and lumpy in appearance. Usually the child will have only a single strawberry haemangioma, usually on the face, neck or trunk, though they can occur anywhere. Occasionally a child will have a number scattered over several parts of the body. Parents often become alarmed at the rapid increase in size over the first six months and are anxious to have it removed. It is only the very occasional child in whom the haemangioma needs to be treated, either by surgical removal or laser therapy, and this is when they are close to vital structures such as the eye or throat, or when they bleed or become infected. However, this is very uncommon and the vast majority do not need any treatment. After the initial surge in growth, they slowly shrivel over time so that by the time the child is nine or ten years of age the haemangioma has disappeared completely.

Port wine stain

These are flat and dark red in colour and are usually present on the face or limbs, often only on one side. They are caused by dilated capillaries (small blood vessels) just under the skin. Unlike strawberry haemangiomas, they do not go away, though sometimes they fade over time. They are problematic only for their appearance, though very rarely a port wine stain on the face can be associated with a structural abnormality of the brain (Sturge-Weber Syndrome). Port wine stains if they are small can be disguised by make-up, though increasingly specialised laser techniques are being used successfully to obliterate them or at least make them much less prominent.

Cradle cap (seborrheic dermatitis)

Cradle cap appears as an oily, crusty or scaly covering on the scalp of an infant in the first year of life, though it can also be present in toddlers. Sometimes it extends to the face and the nappy area.

Cause

It is believed to be due to excessive secretions of the oil glands in the skin, probably stimulated by the mother's hormones which still circulate in the infant's bloodstream for some time after birth.

Signs and symptoms

Cradle cap appears as scaly or crusty patches over the baby's scalp. It is greasy and difficult to peel off, though it does not seem to worry her at all. Sometimes it extends behind the ears and around the neck, armpits and groin area. It can also involve the nappy areas, where it takes on an unsightly, shiny appearance like a very severe nappy rash.

Treatment

The time-honoured treatment is to rub olive oil into the scalp to soften the crusts, which can then be removed at bath time. This may work when the cradle cap is mild or covers a small area of the scalp. More effective are the special shampoos that can be bought at the chemist; these usually clear up the cradle cap in a short period of time. Sometimes a cortisone ointment is necessary to clear up areas elsewhere on the body. The nappy area in particular can become infected with yeast, giving it a red, shiny appearance, and then special preparations will be needed to clear this up.

When to seek medical advice

If the cradle cap cannot be controlled or eradicated with simple remedies as outlined above, and especially if it is getting worse or other areas of the body are affected, then medical advice should be sought. Sometimes cradle cap can be confused with eczema, and the correct diagnosis is important so that appropriate treatment can be obtained.

Eczema

Eczema is a common skin condition in children. It has a genetic contribution so that it tends to run in families, and is associated with asthma, allergies and hay fever. Some have mild eczema or it is transient and the child quickly grows out of it. Others have a more chronic condition which needs virtually constant treatment and sometimes flares up very severely.

Cause

The exact cause of eczema is unknown. It has a genetic basis and runs in families, and it is clear that allergy plays a major role. It is thought that diet is a factor, though it is difficult to pinpoint which foods make it worse. The skin of children with eczema is dry and sensitive, and is easily irritated by chemicals such as harsh detergents and soaps and by contact with woollen or synthetic materials.

Signs and symptoms

Eczema often begins in the first six months of life as a very itchy red rash, usually in patches on the face, and the creases of the elbows and behind the knees. The rash may develop cracks and weep or bleed, and the rest of the skin is very dry. Because it is so itchy, the child will often scratch and rub the skin, which makes it more cracked and can result in the eczema becoming infected. Often the rash will improve as the child gets older, though the skin will remain dry and sensitive. In some children eczema does not appear until the toddler years or later.

Treatment

There are three aspects to the treatment of eczema:

▶ control of dryness;
▶ control of itch; and
▶ treatment of the eczema.

Control of dryness

Children with eczema have dry skin; the drier the skin, the more itchy it becomes and the more likely the child will rub and scratch it, thus increasing the chance of damaging it. Avoid hot baths, which dry the skin. Use bath oils instead of soaps. Use moisturising creams at night after a bath, or as needed several times a day.

Control of itch

Itch is a central feature of eczema, and a major problem. As well as making the child uncomfortable and irritable, scratching makes the eczema worse and increases the chance of infection. Make sure the child's fingernails are cut short. Cotton mittens are often used, especially in the younger child and especially at night. Keep the child's skin cool by avoiding hot baths and avoiding overdressing. Use cotton pyjamas and clothes. Apply moisturising creams liberally.

Treatment of the eczema itself

Treat the rash as soon as it appears. Apart from the moisturising creams, there are a variety of cortisone creams and ointments which are the mainstay of eczema treatment. Ointments are used for dry areas and creams for areas that are moist and weepy. They come in various strengths and formulations, and should be used under close medical supervision. The prolonged and injudicious use of cortisone creams and ointments can themselves cause damage to the skin; on the face especially milder formulations are used to minimise the risk of damage to the skin. If it is suspected that certain foods aggravate the eczema, then a trial omission of these foods from the diet may be worthwhile. This is best done under close supervision by a paediatrician, skin specialist or dietician.

When to seek medical advice

A child with chronic, persistent or recurrent eczema should be under close medical supervision. Medical review is advised if there is a flare-up of the eczema, or if the rash is cracked, weeping or bleeding, or if the child is scratching constantly and appears irritable and distracted.

Prevention

Controlling the dryness and the itch, as outlined above, can go a long way to making the child with eczema more comfortable and avoiding flare-ups. Eczema is not contagious in any way.

Hair loss (alopecia)

It is normal for babies to be born without hair, or to lose some or even all of their hair in the weeks following birth. Hair loss later in childhood is much less common, and not a normal thing to happen.

Cause

The commonest cause of hair loss in children is ringworm (see page 94). Sometimes hair loss can be caused by braids or ponytails that are very tight, and some children, especially girls, may pull out bits of hair due to anxiety or some other emotional upset. There is also a condition called 'alopecia areata', which results in often large patches of hair loss; this tends to be familial, so that there is a genetic component.

Signs and symptoms

Depending on the cause and severity, hair loss can vary from very slight to so significant that bare patches of scalp are visible and the child may be very self-conscious about it. Ringworm may cause other symptoms such as itchiness, and there may be the characteristic features of ringworm present around the area of hair loss.

Treatment

Treatment depends on the underlying cause. There is no treatment for alopecia areata. Often the problem is self-limited.

When to seek medical advice

Any child with hair loss should be seen by a doctor to try to identify the underlying cause.

Head lice (pediculosis)

Head lice is a frequent, often recurring problem which is sometimes wrongly attributed to poor hygiene or unclean personal habits. Perhaps the majority of preschool and school-age children will at some time have head lice, and it is a source of concern and embarrassment to parents, though there are no serious medical consequences. Epidemics of head lice frequently sweep through preschools and schools in all areas of a community.

Cause

Lice are tiny insects about 2–4 mm in size. They lay eggs on the scalp (nits), which take about a week to hatch. They are spread from person to person through close contact or by sharing a comb or a hat. Head lice only survive on humans, and if removed from the head they die very quickly.

Signs and symptoms

The first sign of head lice is an itchy scalp. On close examination, one can see tiny white oval shaped eggs (nits) attached firmly to the base of the hairs, close to the scalp. Sometimes the lice themselves are visible, but the presence of the eggs signifies that the child has head lice.

Treatment

Treatment consists of three separate and important steps. The first step is using a special shampoo available from the chemist to wash the child's hair thoroughly. The shampoo contains a chemical (malathion, lindane or pyrethrin) which kills the lice. The instructions on the bottle must be followed carefully. This treatment is repeated a second time after 7 days to kill any newly hatched eggs.

The second step is to comb out the hair to get rid of the nits, using a special fine-toothed metal comb. This should be done several times following the use of the shampoo. The third step is to wash the pillow case, bed clothes and any hats the child has been wearing in hot water (at least 60° Celcius). Also soak the child's combs and brushes in the anti-lice shampoo for a few hours.

Remember that head lice are very contagious and often recur. This does not mean that the treatment has been unsuccessful. More likely is that there has been re-infection. If the child has head lice it is important that the child care centre or preschool is notified, so that all the children in that setting can be checked and treated if necessary. It is also important to check other members of the family, including adults, for head lice.

When to seek medical advice

Head lice are more of a nuisance than a serious medical problem, and usually it is not necessary to see a doctor.

Prevention

Tying back a girl's long hair may minimise her chances of being infected or re-infected with head lice.

Hives (urticaria)

Hives is an allergic reaction to a variety of substances, which is expressed as a red, very itchy raised rash in the skin. It is quite dramatic in its onset and is very uncomfortable, but rarely serious.

Cause

Hives can be caused by allergies to certain types of foods (cheese, eggs, nuts, shellfish, berries), artificial colourings, medications (penicillin and others), inhaled substances (pollens), bites and stings (bees and other insects), substances that are touched (plants, animals, ointments), and sometimes can be a response to a viral infection. Very often no cause can be found.

Signs and symptoms

Large, white or pinkish-red raised welts appear anywhere on the body but most often on the trunk. Sometimes they may fade and disappear from one area of the body only to reappear in another area, all within a couple of hours. Often they have a whitish centre and are intensely itchy and uncomfortable. The intense phase lasts a few hours, and it then begins to resolve spontaneously.

Treatment

There is little one can do in terms of effective treatment. The itch may be lessened with cool compresses or calamine lotion, and sometimes an antihistamine may help. The best consolation is that the whole episode does not last long, so it is a matter of distracting the child and making her comfortable in the expectation that the rash and itchiness will soon disappear.

When to seek medical advice

Many parents will seek medical advice because of the dramatic onset of hives and the child's discomfort. If the child has any associated breathing difficulties, a hoarse voice or cough, or complains of tightness in the chest then medical advice must be sought as a matter of urgency. (See Allergic reactions, page 18.)

Prevention

If hives recur at regular intervals, sometimes the cause can be identified and then efforts made to avoid it.

Impetigo (school sores)

Impetigo is a bacterial skin infection seen commonly in preschool and school age-children; it is very contagious.

Cause

Impetigo is usually caused by one of two bacteria — streptococcus, which is also the cause of some cases of tonsillitis, or staphylococcus. Occasionally there is an underlying skin condition such as scabies or eczema where the skin is broken down and so there is a predisposition to infection.

Signs and symptoms

Sores can appear anywhere on the body, but are commonest on the face (around the nose, mouth and ears), and also on the hands, arms and legs. They begin as small red spots that grow in size and turn into blisters which in time break and ooze a yellow thick fluid and which then tend to form scabs. Sometimes no blisters are evident but crusts and yellowish scabs are formed. They are usually itchy and the child scratches at them. This results in pulling off the scabs and spreading the infection to surrounding areas or to other parts of the body. Often the lymph glands in adjacent areas (neck, groin or armpit) are swollen and may be tender.

Treatment

The sores are bathed with warm water and soap and the crusts lifted gently off. If there are only one or two spots, an antibiotic or antiseptic cream is applied several times a day, and the area is covered if possible (this is difficult if the sores are on the face) to prevent the spread of infection to other parts of the body and to other children. If there are widespread areas of sores, or if the infection is more extensive, the child is given antibiotics to be taken by mouth. These days it is usual for antibiotics to be given to hasten resolution and to make sure that they do not spread.

Because they are so infectious, the child with impetigo is excluded from the early childhood setting unless the sores can be entirely covered or until they heal.

When to seek medical advice

It is a good idea to have a doctor assess the child unless the sores are very small and isolated and if parents are sure that they are impetigo. If they are spreading, or are present across several areas of the body, then prescription medicines are usually necessary and the child needs to be seen by a doctor.

Prevention

Because school sores can spread so quickly, where possible they should be covered. A child with extensive school sores or where it is not possible to cover them up should be kept home until healing is well underway; that is until there are no scabs or ooze from existing sores. Keep a separate towel for exclusive use of the child with impetigo. Make sure her nails are cut short and discourage scratching and picking at the scabs. (See also Exclusion Table, page 79.)

Nappy rash

Nappy rash refers to a rash or irritation in the ano-genital area that is covered by a nappy. It is very common in infants and toddlers before they are toilet-trained, and may occur despite the most careful attention and good hygiene.

Cause

Sometimes nappy rash is referred to as 'irritant napkin dermatitis', as it is really an inflammation of the nappy area caused by prolonged contact with and reaction to urine and faeces. Ammonia is released from the urine and this further irritates the skin. Plastic pants may make the situation worse as they do not allow air to get to the skin. Once the surface of the skin is damaged, it becomes even more vulnerable to the effects of prolonged contact with urine and faeces. If the child has diarrhoea for several days, this may result in a nappy rash.

Sometimes seborrheic dermatitis (see page 83) causes a rash in the nappy area, and in some infants there is a secondary yeast infection (candida albicans or thrush).

Signs and symptoms

The first sign of nappy rash is usually redness or small bumps in the area of skin covered by the nappy. Some areas may progress to ulceration of the skin. The skin folds are usually not involved as they are protected from direct contact with urine or faeces.

If the rash is seborrheic dermatitis, it presents as a red scaly rash with the skin creases of the groin involved. Where there is secondary yeast infection, the nappy areas look red and shiny, and spots (satellite lesions) may be scattered beyond the outer edge of the rash.

Nappy rash may be uncomfortable for the infant or young child and, if the inflammation is severe or there is ulceration of the skin, may cause pain. He may therefore be irritable and unsettled.

Treatment

The nappy area should be kept clean and dry. A wet or dirty nappy should be changed as soon as possible to minimise contact with the skin. Ideally the nappy should be checked every hour or so, at least during the day time hours. Whenever possible and practical, the nappy should be left off completely to allow contact with air. When the nappy is changed, the ano-genital area should be washed gently with warm water and a mild soap, and carefully dried. A protective cream should be used after each nappy change. These usually have a zinc base and can be bought over the counter from the chemist.

If seborrheic dermatitis or yeast infection are present, these are treated with specific creams or ointments prescribed by the doctor.

When to seek medical advice

Simple nappy rashes do not need medical assessment — treatment is as outlined above. When the nappy rash is severe and not responding to these simple measures, or if the skin is ulcerated and causing distress to the child, or if there are features suggesting seborrheoic dermatitis or yeast infection (see above), then the child should be seen by a doctor.

Prevention

The simple measures outlined above, if used consistently, should help prevent nappy rash or, if it does occur, to clear it up quickly.

Ringworm

Ringworm is a fungal infection contracted from infected cats or dogs, and which causes characteristic lesions on the skin or scalp. It has nothing to do with worms.

Cause

Ringworm is contracted directly from the animals and then spread from person to person by direct contact or by sharing combs and hairbrushes. When a child with ringworm touches or scratches the rash, the fungus sticks to the fingers or gets under the fingernails and spreads when the child touches someone else.

Signs and symptoms

Ringworm appears as a scaly, red circular patch on the trunk or on the scalp. Usually there is only a single patch. Initially it looks like a red patch with a raised or lumpy edge. It is only later as the patch grows that the centre of it becomes more clear in colour and the whole lesion takes on the appearance of a ring. After some weeks the patch stops growing, but others may form nearby so that there is a cluster, but still usually in the same area.

If the lesion is in the scalp, there are one or more patches of hair loss with some short, dull hairs present there rather than the normal longer healthy hair. Redness and scaling is present on the scalp at the base.

Treatment

Ringworm usually responds to treatment with anti-fungal creams, though it may take some time to clear up completely. If the lesions persist and do not seem to respond to treatment, or if it is ringworm of the scalp, then a course of medication to be taken by mouth is often necessary.

When to seek medical advice

The diagnosis of ringworm is usually made by observing the pattern of the lesions on the scalp or body as described above, but sometimes a special light is used (Wood's lamp); the lesions of ringworm have a characteristic glow under this light.

Prevention

Pet animals that have bare patches in their fur or coats where the hair looks brittle and has fallen out leaving short stumps may have ringworm and should be treated by the vet. This may prevent spread to children. Children infected with ringworm should be excluded from child care or preschool until treatment has commenced, unless the lesion can be covered. (See also Exclusion Table, page 79.)

Scabies

Scabies is an infection of the skin by a tiny insect or mite that causes an intensely itchy rash. It is highly contagious, and often occurs in outbreaks in preschools and schools.

Cause

Scabies is caused by a microscopic mite which burrows into the skin and lays its eggs in tunnels just below the surface of the skin. Once the mite gets into the skin, it takes 2–6 weeks for the rash to appear. Scabies is spread from child to child by touch or by contact with infected clothing or other personal items.

Signs and symptoms

The rash appears as numerous red lumps and thread-like tracks, especially between the fingers and toes, on the insides of the wrists, in the groin region and on the buttocks. The rash is intensely itchy, and the child will be constantly scratching it. The itch seems worse after a hot bath and at night time. Sometimes the constant scratching leads to secondary infection.

Treatment

The whole family needs to be treated, and the child kept at home until treatment has been successful. The early childhood setting should be notified so all affected children and their families can be treated. Re-infection after treatment is not uncommon.

The definitive treatment is a special lotion that is prescribed by the doctor, and is applied to the whole body (except the face) after a hot bath. It is left on for at least 8 hours before being washed off. All family members should be treated at the same time, and the child's clothing and bed linen should be washed. The itch may still take another week or two after this treatment before it settles — this does not mean that the treatment has been unsuccessful. Calamine lotion and sometimes an antihistamine may relieve the itch.

When to seek medical advice

If scabies is suspected because of the intense itch and rash, or because someone else in the family or child care or preschool setting has it, a doctor should be consulted to confirm the diagnosis and to prescribe the specific treatment. Sometimes the scabies becomes infected as a result of the scratching, and then this also needs to be checked and treated by the doctor.

Prevention

The initial infection cannot be prevented. To prevent the spread of scabies, all the family members should be treated at the same time, and clothes and linen and soft toys washed. The child should be kept at home until the treatment has been applied. (See also Exclusion Table, page 79.)

Sunburn/sun protection

Protection from the sun and avoidance of sunburn is a major public health issue in Australia. Young children have very sensitive skin which is easily burned. Australia has one of the highest rates of skin cancers in the world, and there is evidence that this may be due at least in part to early excessive exposure to the sun.

Cause

The skin contains a pigment called melanin, which serves to protect it from the rays of the sun. People with an olive or dark skin have more melanin in their skin than fair people, and therefore have more protection from the sun. If exposure to the sun is gradual, then more melanin is produced and the skin tans. Where exposure is sudden or excessive, there has not been time for melanin to be produced or else there is not enough to afford protection, and sunburn results.

Signs and symptoms

Sunburn can vary from mild redness of the skin to marked blistering. It can cause mild discomfort through to severe pain.

Treatment

Severe sunburn is treated like any other burn (see page 24). Where the sunburn is mild, the child can be made more comfortable by wearing loose clothing or no clothing at all if the room is warm. Make sure she drinks lots, and paracetamol can be given for pain.

When to seek medical advice

If there are blisters present, or if the skin has broken and is weeping, or if the pain is severe, then medical assessment and advice should be obtained.

Prevention

The skin of young children is especially sensitive to the sun. Community early childhood settings such as child care, preschool and schools should be designed with protection from the sun in mind. Outdoor play areas should be shaded by trees, verandas and shade cloth. Try to avoid outdoor activities in the middle of the day when the sun is hottest, and then make sure the children wear suitable protective clothing — hats and long sleeves — and apply sunblock to exposed areas.

Warts

Warts are common in children over the age of two years. They may cause embarrassment but are not serious and usually resolve over time without treatment.

Cause

There are several types of warts, all caused by an infection with a virus (human papilloma virus). They spread by direct skin contact from one area to another in the same child, and from one child to another.

Signs and symptoms

Warts appear gradually and are painless. The common wart grows on the hands, elbows and knees. Another type of wart seems to appear in crops on the face and hands, and are called plane warts. Warts that grow on the soles of the feet are called plantar warts; these can cause pain and discomfort if they are on weight bearing areas. Warts may be embarrassing for the child, especially older children, and this is the main indication for treatment.

Treatment

Most warts will disappear in time without any treatment. If they are unsightly, there are special preparations that can be purchased from the chemist which are painted on the warts. These soften the heaped up skin of the wart which can then be picked off using a fingernail or nail file. A plantar wart which is causing pain and discomfort can also be treated in this way but, because it is larger, needs medical supervision and usually a stronger preparation. Sometimes the warts can be burnt off or removed surgically, but this should be avoided if possible as they can still recur and may result in scarring.

When to seek medical advice

If the warts are extensive and present on the face, or if a plantar wart is causing pain or discomfort and interfering with walking and running, then the child should be seen by a doctor, who can initiate appropriate treatment.

Prevention

Warts are contagious, and picking at them will serve to spread them to different parts of the body. Wearing rubber thongs in public places such as swimming pools and showers will lessen the chance of the child picking up the virus and causing a plantar wart.

Genitourinary
Foreskin and circumcision

While for a long time circumcision was the norm for the majority of boys, over recent years it has lost its popularity. These days it is a minority of boys who are circumcised in the neonatal period. While for some religions and ethnic groups ritual circumcision is routine, more parents are deciding against circumcising their male infants.

Arguments are put forward for and against circumcision, but from a medical point of view these pretty much balance each other out, so in the end it is parental preference rather than any medical reasoning one way or the other.

When the foreskin remains, there are anatomical issues parents and professionals should be aware of, together with some problems that might arise.

In young boys the foreskin covering the glans (head) of the penis is firmly attached and cannot be fully retracted until the boy is 4–5 years of age. The foreskin should never be forcibly retracted.

Sometimes the foreskin can become inflamed (balanitis) and, occasionally, if this is recurrent, partial or complete circumcision may be necessary. Phimosis is when the opening of the foreskin is very small, and in severe cases may interfere with passing urine.

Mostly these problems will not be the concern of early childhood professionals, and if any action or special care is needed on their part then parents will discuss these with them.

Enuresis (wetting)

Wetting at night is called nocturnal enuresis, though strictly speaking the wetting can occur whenever the child is asleep, and can include wetting when the child has a day time sleep. There is considerable variability in the time children are toilet-trained, but about 10–15% of children are still wetting the bed when they start school. A diagnosis of enuresis is only made in children older than four years of age. Any younger than this and it is considered simply that the child is not yet toilet-trained.

Cause

Despite the still commonly held belief that enuresis is behavioural or psychological, research now suggests that it is genetic in origin (so it frequently runs in families), and is due to an arousal disorder so the child when asleep is unresponsive to the sensation of bladder fullness. There may also be a deficiency of the hormone that normally concentrates the urine at night time (anti-diuretic hormone or ADH). Very occasionally psychological upset may play a role in a child who has been dry and then begins to wet again. However, if there are psychological disturbances in children with nocturnal enuresis, they are usually secondary to the wetting and resolve once the wetting is cured. Very occasionally bedwetting may be due to other causes such as a urinary infection.

Signs and symptoms

Some children wet every night, and sometimes more than once during the night. Others wet several times a week, or less frequently. They wake up in a wet bed either during the night or in the morning. Some children wake up while they are urinating, and then are able to go to the toilet to finish. However, most children sleep right through the episode. The child reacts with varying degrees of embarrassment or feigned indifference, depending on her age and the reactions of her family to the wetting. Older children inevitably suffer a loss of self-esteem and their wetting will interfere with other aspects of their lives and with their peer relationships. For example, they will be reluctant to sleep over at a friend's house or to go on school camps. It is a condition that is often distressing for child and parents alike.

Treatment

It is generally accepted that treatment should not begin before the age of 4–5 years; until they start school is a good rule of thumb. Up until that age bedwetting can be regarded as still within the range of normal maturation.

If no treatment is offered, about 15% get better each year. However, by the time children get to school age, it is likely that it will increasingly have an effect on the child's self-esteem and daily life, so treatment is recommended unless the wetting is infrequent and clearly not having negative consequences on the child or family.

There are a variety of interventions that can be tried, though the results are not very good or sustainable, and do not cure the problem. These include restricting the amount of fluid the child drinks in the evening, the parents waking the child and taking her to the toilet during the night, and the use of star charts and other behavioural incentives.

The usual first line of treatment is the use of an alarm. This can be hired from a clinic at a children's hospital, from some pharmacies, and from continence services in the community. It is best if its use is on the advice and under the supervision of a doctor. The average course of treatment is 6–8 weeks, and it will cure between two-thirds and three-quarters of children. Some relapse after apparent cure, but then respond to a second course of treatment.

Where the child has not responded to two attempts with the alarm, then a hormone (ADH) nasal spray is prescribed and is taken in the evening just before bedtime (this should be under the supervision of a paediatrician). It has the effect of concentrating the urine and making it less likely the child will have a full bladder during the night.

It goes without saying that the child should never be scolded or punished for wetting the bed, as it is totally outside her control. Carers and teachers should help the child change her clothes with a minimum of fuss when she has wet.

When to seek medical advice

It is a good idea to ask the doctor to help with the management of bedwetting.

Day time wetting

Day time wetting is usually more distressing and embarrassing than bedwetting because it occurs during the day and is noticeable by other children, though many children who do wet during the day seem oblivious to it.

Cause

The most common reason for children to wet during the day, especially in early childhood settings, is that they are not fully toilet-trained. A number of preschool children who have already been toilet-trained will still wet occasionally during the day, especially if they are busy playing, or during a nap. However there are other reasons why children wet during the day — these can include anatomical and functional problems with the bladder and the muscles surrounding its base; lack of coordination between the bladder neck and surrounding muscles so that bladder emptying is incomplete and urine that remains continues to leak out into the child's underpants; neurological problems that interfere with bladder function; or urinary infections. Day time wetting can be part of the spectrum of emotional upset in some children, while others seem to become so involved and preoccupied with activities that they do not seem to feel the urge to go to the toilet, or if they do feel it they often simply ignore it.

Signs and symptoms

This varies with the cause. Some children will saturate their clothes with urine, while others will have small wet patches on their underwear. Some will wet occasionally, while others will seemingly be wet all or most of the time. Sometimes the child will not be aware that she has wet, even though it is apparent to others who can smell the urine as well as notice the wet clothes. Other children, especially the older ones, will be embarrassed and this may affect their confidence and their social relationships. Most children will wet during the day from early childhood — that is they have never been really dry during the day, while others begin day time wetting after a variable period of being dry.

Treatment

Again this depends on the cause. It may involve use of medication, and many of these children will need investigations including special X-rays and sometimes cystoscopy (in which the paediatric surgeon passes an instrument into the bladder). Most children with day time wetting, whatever the cause, will need a structured behavioural and toiletting regime. This means being taken to the toilet at specified intervals, often the use of a diary, rewards for staying dry, and so on. Early childhood professionals are often essential members of the team and their cooperation is crucial if the child's management is to be successful.

When to seek medical advice

Any child who is said to be fully toilet-trained and wets during the day should be seen by a doctor and may need further specialist referral to a paediatrician.

Haematuria (blood in the urine)

This is uncommon in young children, but when it occurs always needs to be taken seriously and investigated.

Cause

The most common cause is an infection of the urinary tract. Other causes include physical injury, kidney inflammation, or a bleeding disorder.

Signs and symptoms

The child's urine has a red, orange or brown colour. Depending on the cause, there may be some pain or burning on urination, or discomfort in the kidney area, or no symptoms at all. More common is that frank blood in the urine is what is called 'microscopic haematuria' — small traces of blood that are only seen under a microscope or by testing the urine with a chemical reagent.

Treatment

This depends on the cause. Infection is treated with antibiotics (see Urinary tract infection, page 107). Investigations are always needed to identify the cause of the bleeding.

When to seek medical advice

The child who is suspected of having blood in her urine should always be seen by a doctor as soon as possible to establish the cause and institute appropriate treatment.

Toilet-training

Toilet-training can be the easiest or most difficult of milestones for young children to achieve. It is something that many parents worry about. Some early childhood settings insist on the child being trained as a condition of enrolment and attendance, and by the time the child begins school he is well and truly expected to be trained. However, in younger children, early childhood professionals may well find themselves not only supporting the parents as they attempt to train the child, but often being very much involved themselves in helping to train him.

Toilet-training is understandably thought of as a very important milestone for parents. It is such a visible and concrete achievement for their young child, and inevitably there will be comparison and even competition with friends' children. There may be additional pressure from grandparents or the need for the child to be trained before beginning preschool.

The timing of a child being fully trained and whether it is easy or difficult depends on a number of factors. The child needs to be physically, neurologically and emotionally ready. This means there is little point even thinking of beginning training before the child's second birthday. The child's temperament is also a factor, as is his relationship with the parents and their parenting style. Toilet-training usually begins at the age when the child is going through the developmental stage of establishing some independence from the parents, with the attendant testing of limits and temper tantrums. Trying to train the child at this time can easily end up as a power struggle between the child and parents.

For some children toilet-training is a non-event, with everything going very smoothly and the child becoming fully trained in a short period of time. In others it can take ages and be traumatic for child and parents alike. Despite the considerable individual variation, most children are trained during the day time at least by 3–4 years, and at night by the time they begin school. The usual sequence is that the child first achieves bowel continence, and then urinary continence, first during the day and then at night.

The role of the early childhood professional

Parents may seek advice or reassurance about when and how to toilet-train the child, especially if they are under pressure from the centre or preschool to have their child continent. It would be useful to have available some parent information, or to be able to direct them to a credible book or, if they are having difficulty, to suggest they speak to their paediatrician or interested general practitioner.

Often parents will have begun to train the child at home, and the early childhood professional will be asked to participate and continue the training regime in the early childhood setting. Depending on the age of the child and the way the parents have gone about the training, early childhood professionals may be asked to take the child to the toilet or put him on a potty at set times, or ask the child from time to time whether he needs to go to the toilet, or respond to his body language or other clues. If he has an accident, he will need to be cleaned up and changed with a minimum of fuss. It goes without saying that the child should never be punished for having an accident while he is being toilet-trained.

The best results will be achieved where the professionals and parents work closely in partnership, and are clear about expectations and exactly what to do. It makes sense for the same routines to be used at home and at the centre or preschool, and for there to be agreement about strategies to be used, the nature and timing of prompts, the type of reward and reinforcement the child responds to, and so on.

Where the child and/or parents are becoming stressed by the training, or where other difficulties are encountered, the provision of appropriate advice can be very important. If the problem is perceived to be severe, or where advice is felt to be beyond the expertise and confidence of the carer or teacher, then referral for professional help is indicated.

The child who is 'difficult' to toilet-train

With some children, toilet-training is very difficult. There are a number of reasons for this. Some children are developmentally delayed, so even if they are at the chronological age where most children will achieve continence, in fact developmentally they are functioning at a younger age. Others may have a physical condition such as cerebral palsy, constipation or chronic diarrhoea.

Many children become so engrossed in play activities that they literally 'forget' to go to the toilet — they simply do not pay heed to the signals of a full bladder until it is too late. These children may take longer to train completely; often there is a pattern of occasional wetting, usually of small amounts, when they are busy with the daily activities of the setting. Early childhood professionals have an important role to play by reminding children to go to the toilet regularly, or scheduling it as part of their daily routine.

A number of children seem resistant to being trained as a consequence of the relationship they have with the parents. Whatever the characteristics of the child and the parents, there is a power struggle going on so that the more the parents try the more the child resists. Often the parents may benefit from guidance provided by their family doctor or paediatrician.

Urinary tract infection

Urinary tract infections are relatively common in young children, especially in girls.

Cause

Infections of the bladder or kidneys are caused by bacteria and always need treatment with appropriate antibiotics. In about 40% of cases there is an underlying anatomical abnormality which predisposes the child to infection and, if unrecognised, will lead to recurrent infections.

Signs and symptoms

Very young children may have vague and non-specific symptoms such as fever, poor weight gain, irritability or vomiting. Older children will have the classic and well recognised features such as burning or scalding when passing urine, a frequent urge to urinate, and sometimes wetting during the day or night when the child has previously been dry. Sometimes the urine is concentrated and smelly, and occasionally bloody or dark in colour. Older children may also have accompanying fever, poor appetite, and sometimes loin pain if the infection is in the kidney. Some children are very sick with a urinary infection, while others may be mildly ill.

Treatment

Children under the age of 12 months and those who are sick will need to be admitted to hospital, at least initially. Older children are given antibiotics to take by mouth, usually for 5–7 days or until there is laboratory proof that the infection has cleared up. All children with a confirmed urinary tract infection need to have special X-rays of their kidneys and urinary tract to see if there are underlying anatomical abnormalities. If these are present, and depending on their nature, some children will need to take a small daily dose of antibiotics to prevent a recurrence of infection. Some young children will need to take medication for years, others for months. Occasionally surgery is necessary to correct the abnormality.

When to seek medical advice

If a urinary tract infection is suspected, it is essential the child be seen by a doctor so that an accurate diagnosis can be made, appropriate treatment implemented, and follow up with X-rays organised. Even if the symptoms suggest an infection, it is essential to check a clean fresh sample of urine to confirm the diagnosis and to identify the bacteria which is responsible. This helps the doctor choose the best antibiotic.

Gastrointestinal

Abdominal pain

Abdominal pain is common in young children. Mostly it is not serious and passes quickly with no treatment. Occasionally urgent medical assessment and treatment is required.

Causes

There are many causes of abdominal pain; these vary according to the age of the child.

In the younger child the pain can be due to gastroenteritis (page 123) or to constipation (page 113) or rarely to a condition caused intussusception in which a part of the small intestine telescopes or slides into itself and causes a bowel obstruction. Sometimes 'colic' in infants (page 176) is said to be due to abdominal pain because of the crying and often drawing up of the legs, though there is no evidence that this is the case.

In older children, gastroenteritis is still perhaps the commonest cause of acute abdominal pain, but other causes need also to be considered. Constipation is relatively common, and appendicitis is the commonest surgical cause of acute abdominal pain. Pain may occur with any viral infection, presumably due to inflammation of lymph glands and lymphoid tissue around the intestines. Migraine (page 143) in children manifests itself as abdominal pain, which at times is more prominent than the classical headaches normally associated with this condition and seen in adults. Urinary tract infection (page 107) may be associated with abdominal pain, and food poisoning will often cause pain along with diarrhoea and vomiting. Finally, some children seem to have recurrent abdominal pain in response to anxiety and stress.

Signs and symptoms

The nature of the abdominal pain depends on the cause. It can be sharp and acute or a dull ache. It can come in spasms so it comes on and then disappears quickly, or may be constant. The abdominal pain may be the only symptom, or there may be other gastrointestinal symptoms such as nausea, vomiting, and diarrhoea present as well.

In gastroenteritis and food poisoning, there is always diarrhoea and often vomiting, and the pain is acute and sharp and comes on suddenly. With intussusception, the child looks pale and quite sick, the pain comes in spasms, and usually there is the passage of stool with blood in it (called redcurrant stool). Children with pain associated with a viral infection will have typical symptoms. The pain associated with constipation is often colicky in nature, comes and goes, and is sometimes relieved by the child having a bowel movement. In urinary infection, the pain is usually present when passing urine, but infections of the kidney will cause a dull ache in the loin and back area. The pain of appendicitis is sharp and constant, beginning often in the middle of the stomach around the belly button and then moving down to the lower right side of the abdomen. Migraine is associated with nausea and vomiting and often headache, while stress and anxiety causes a vague dull pain that is usually in the centre of the abdomen, but is often difficult for the child to localise.

The pain is usually more likely to be serious if it wakes the child from sleep or is in a specific area of the abdomen away from the belly button.

When to seek medical advice

Children with abdominal pain should always be seen by a doctor to rule out appendicitis or another medical condition that needs urgent treatment. Most children with abdominal pain will turn out to have something that is transient and not serious, but it is not always easy to know this without taking a careful history and conducting a thorough physical examination.

Appendicitis

Appendicitis is a fairly common condition in childhood and always requires surgical intervention.

Cause

Appendicitis is caused by inflammation of the appendix, a small blind finger-like protrusion of the large bowel. The appendix serves no known function. It is not known why the appendix suddenly becomes inflamed, except sometimes it may get blocked by a hard piece of faeces called a faecolith. The inflammation causes the appendix to swell, and if not removed it may burst and cause peritonitis, which is an inflammation of the lining of the intestines. This is a serious and sometimes even fatal condition, and is one reason why urgent surgical attention is important in cases of acute appendicitis.

Signs and symptoms

Appendicitis usually begins as a dull pain in the middle of the abdomen, and after a few hours usually moves to the right side of the body and becomes sharper and more severe. The child may feel nauseated and generally unwell, and even vomit. Fever may be present, and the child will not be hungry. Gradually the pain increases in intensity, so that the child will be reluctant to walk and may stoop over; any movement makes the pain worse.

Treatment

The treatment of acute appendicitis is surgical removal. This necessitates admission to hospital for a few days, but most children are back to their normal everyday activities in a very short period of time.

When to seek medical advice

If appendicitis is suspected, then the child must be seen by a doctor without delay. Indeed, any child with severe abdominal pain of acute onset must have urgent medical attention. Appendicitis usually presents with classic signs and symptoms, as described above, in which case diagnosis is straightforward. However it can also be very difficult to diagnose.

Breastfeeding

'Breast is best' is a common saying which underscores the fact that breastfeeding is the best way to feed young infants. Breast milk is convenient, is always at the right temperature, needs no special equipment, and is perfectly nutritionally balanced.

There are other benefits for both mother and baby. Breastfeeding helps cement the intense bond between mother and her baby, and the process of breastfeeding is something that breastfeeding mothers regard as very special. The breastfed infant receives antibodies in the mother's milk which help to protect her against common infectious diseases such as gastroenteritis, and her bowel movements are more likely to be soft and non-offensive. There is recent research suggesting that breastfed infants do better on tests of intelligence as they become older.

For some mothers, breastfeeding is easy and very straightforward; while for others it is a frustrating and often very difficult task. Lots of things can go wrong, including breast infections (mastitis), cracked nipples and an erratic milk supply. Some mothers give up in frustration, but most of these difficulties can be overcome if the mother is determined to breastfeed. Often they are wrongly advised to wean the baby as soon as problems are encountered. Other women give up breastfeeding when they go back to work, wrongly believing that they cannot continue to breastfeed while their child is in care.

The role of the early childhood centre in promoting breastfeeding

Early childhood staff have an important role in encouraging breastfeeding. Mothers can express and store breast milk in a bottle in the fridge. While the child is at the centre he is given expressed breast milk via a bottle, but sucks at the breast when he is with his mother. This option can be offered to all breastfeeding mothers who utilise child care. If the mother is having difficulties breastfeeding, child care staff can suggest a referral to a community nurse, lactation consultant or doctor, or to the Australian Breastfeeding Association. Their website address is <**http://www.breastfeeding.asn.au**> and they have helpline numbers in each state and territory.

Bottle feeding

Some mothers are unable or choose not to breastfeed, or wean the baby at early age. They should be supported in this decision once it is made, and should not be made to feel guilty. Modern formulae are specially constituted to closely mimic breastmilk. Sometimes already made up formula will be left at the centre for the child, and staff simply have to heat it up, or they will need to make up the formula. This should be done closely following the instructions on the can, and scrupulous cleanliness is essential. Staff should wash their hands before preparing the bottle, and the milk should be warmed in the microwave or a jug of hot water. If a microwave is used, care needs to be taken as the milk may have warmed unevenly and may be too hot. Prepared formula should be stored in the refrigerator until it is time for it to be given to the child.

Constipation

The frequency of bowel movements varies considerably from child to child, and just because a child goes for a few days without a bowel movement does not mean he is constipated. Constipation is therefore difficult to define, and the definition should not rest only on the frequency of bowel movements. Constipation is best considered to be when the stools become hard and difficult to pass, often with a reduction in the child's usual frequency of passing bowel movements.

Cause

Many factors can contribute to constipation. Dietary factors, especially the lack of water, fibre and roughage, are common contributing factors. Some children hold back from going to the toilet, especially if they are too busy playing or otherwise preoccupied, while toddlers may resist opening their bowels during attempts at toilet-training. Constipation and consequent painful bowel movements in turn lead to the child resisting passing a bowel movement because of the anticipated pain, so creating a cycle which makes matters worse. In some infants and toddlers, the passage of a hard bowel motion causes a small tear in the lining of the anus (anal fissure), making defecation even more painful. Constipation is more common in bottlefed than breastfed infants, and there is a tendency for it to run in families.

Signs and symptoms

Bowel movements are compact, hard and often difficult and painful to pass. There may be a reduction in the child's usual frequency of opening his bowels. There may be associated crampy or vague abdominal pain which sometimes is relieved following a bowel movement. Older children with marked constipation are often described by their parents as being sluggish and as not having much appetite. If an anal fissure is present there may be blood on the nappy or the stool or the toilet paper.

Treatment

The cornerstone of treatment of constipation is dietary. Simply put, the child's diet is modified to increase the amount of fibre. This is achieved by increasing the amount of foods containing fibre and roughage — fruit and vegetables, rice and pasta, high fibre cereals and breads, and dried fruits. It is important to ensure the child is drinking lots of fluids (apart from milk). Older children should be encouraged to sit on the toilet regularly, and sometimes a structured toiletting regime is useful — the child sits on the toilet three times a day at a regular time (usually after a meal) whether or not he feels he needs to go.

Sometimes medicines are used to treat constipation. These are to be considered a short-term solution. They can break the cycle by ensuring the stool is soft and thus make it less likely to be painful, so that the child then has no reason to hold back. In the long term, however, it is the change in the child's diet and regular sitting on the toilet that will make the difference. Early childhood professionals may assist in a management regime by encouraging regular toilet habits.

When to seek medical advice

If the constipation does not improve quickly with the simple measures outlined above, or if there is blood in the stools, or if there is associated abdominal pain, then the child should be assessed by a doctor. Similarly, if the child, especially in the toddler age group, is actively holding back, a behavioural management regime may need to be implemented.

Prevention

The best way to prevent constipation is to ensure the child has a balanced diet, and in older children to ensure they sit on the toilet regularly.

Diarrhoea

Diarrhoea is common in young children. While usually not serious, in very young children especially there is the risk of dehydration so that early assessment and treatment is important. Some children have diarrhoea that is more chronic and persistent.

Cause

There are a number of causes of diarrhoea in children. Often a child will have a day or two of loose stools with no other symptoms, with a rapid return to normal bowel patterns. This is considered to be normal and is no cause for concern. Gastroenteritis (see page 123) is the commonest cause of diarrhoea. Occasionally it is caused by a bacterial or parasitic infection, food poisoning or food allergy. Antibiotics that the child is taking can cause loose stools, as can a generalised viral infection; like vomiting, diarrhoea can accompany many infections.

Chronic diarrhoea is caused most commonly by a temporary lactose (sugar) intolerance that follows gastroenteritis. The lining of the intestine is damaged so it cannot absorb lactose, which then causes the diarrhoea. Excessive consumption of fruit juices, especially apple juice, can cause persistent diarrhoea, and occasionally it may be due to a parasitic infection (giardia) or a manifestation of a more serious condition such as coeliac disease.

Signs and symptoms

Each child's pattern of bowel movements is different. Diarrhoea is considered to be present when the child's bowel movements increase in frequency or change to an unformed watery consistency. There is huge variation in the size and frequency of stools. They may be thin and watery or semi-formed, often offensive, and vary in colour from green to dark brown to a pale colour. Depending on the cause, there may be vomiting and fever, as well as signs of a generalised viral infection. Occasionally there may be associated abdominal pain.

Treatment

The single most important thing is to make sure that the child drinks sufficiently to compensate for the fluids lost in the diarrhoea in addition to her daily needs. If the child is still being breastfed, this should be continued and extra fluids given in the form of oral rehydration fluid. This is made up by adding water to the sachets of powder which are obtained from the chemist (*Gastrolyte; Pedialyte; Repalyte*). In older children and those who are bottle fed, the milk is diluted with water and oral rehydration fluid also given. If the child is hungry and not vomiting, there is no need to withhold solid food but it should be kept bland. If the child is vomiting as well, small amounts of fluids are given frequently rather than large amounts which are less likely to be tolerated.

Medicines to stop or reduce the diarrhoea should never be given to children. They are not effective and can make the condition worse. The child with diarrhoea should be excluded from child care or preschool until the bowel movements have returned to normal.

When to seek medical advice

Young children with severe (5–6 watery stools per day) or persistent diarrhoea should always be checked by a doctor, especially if they are also vomiting and cannot keep anything down or are showing signs of dehydration (see page 117).

Prevention

Diarrhoea is easily spread from person to person in an early childhood setting. Careful attention to hygiene is very important in order to prevent the spread of infection. (See also Exclusion Table, page 79.)

Dehydration

A young child can become dehydrated either because of excessive fluid loss, for example if she has diarrhoea and/or vomiting, or else because of insufficient intake of fluids, for example if she is sick and unable or unwilling to drink.

Cause

Gastroenteritis (page 123) is by far the commonest cause of dehydration in young children. However, any illness which results in persistent diarrhoea, vomiting or reduced fluid intake can lead to dehydration, especially in younger children who have less reserve.

Signs and symptoms

Apart from the features of the illness itself, the child passes less urine or has fewer wet nappies, her tongue and mouth look dry and coated, her eyes will look dark and sunken, and she will look pale and be tired and lethargic. She will have lost weight because of the loss of fluid.

Treatment

Many children become mildly dehydrated during the course of an illness, and recover quickly as they get better without needing any special treatment. Simply increasing the amount of fluid intake for children with fever or a viral illness is all most children require. Oral rehydration fluid is especially effective in gastroenteritis, but can be given to children who are dehydrated for other reasons as well. Very uncommonly the child is so severely dehydrated that she needs admission to hospital for intravenous fluids.

Prevention

Care should be taken to make sure that all children with a viral illness or fever or gastroenteritis drink extra fluids, even if they do not have an appetite.

Encopresis (soiling)

Encopresis refers to the involuntary passage of bowel movements into a place other than the toilet (usually the underpants). The term is used in children over the age of four years; under this age not all children will have been toilet-trained. Some children have an occasional episode of soiling, when they have diarrhoea or do not make it to the toilet in time. It is only when it occurs frequently in children over four years of age that it is considered abnormal. It is much more common in boys.

Cause

The vast majority of children with soiling have underlying retention of faeces. This is different from constipation (see page 113). These children may well have daily bowel movements of normal consistency. However, for a variety of reasons, there is accumulated faeces in the child's rectum and large bowel. This stretches the walls of the bowel, and thus diminishes the sensation of needing to go to the toilet. The signal to the brain for a child of needing to open his bowels is the result of the walls of the bowel stretching in response to the presence of faeces. Because the walls are already stretched due to the accumulation of faeces, the child is not aware of the urge to open his bowels.

Signs and symptoms

There is considerable variation in the pattern of soiling. Some children soil several times a week, while others soil several times a day. Sometimes they are large bowel movements, at other times small amounts or staining (streaking) of the underwear. Some children may go for weeks without soiling, and others may not have a single day without an accident.

Most children have no sensation of needing to go to the toilet, and some are not even aware that they have soiled; they will be oblivious to the smell. Others may have some sensation but do not make it to the toilet in time.

Children will react differently to the soiling. Some will seem totally unaware of what has happened and seem to be indifferent to it. Many will feel shame and embarrassment, especially older children who may be subject to teasing and ridicule from their peers.

Treatment

The best results are achieved using a number of strategies in combination. First is to ensure the child has a well balanced diet, with sufficient fibre and lots of fluids. A poor diet is considered to be one of the reasons the child accumulates faeces in his bowel in the first place. Second is to make sure the child sits on the toilet at regular intervals, especially in the period following a meal. This is something that professionals may be asked to cooperate with. Even if the child has no urge, he sits on the toilet for five minutes or more and attempts to pass a bowel movement. Sometimes a star chart and diary encourages the child to sit regularly. Finally some children need to take medications, at least for an initial period, to assist with evacuation of the retained faeces. These consist either of stool softeners or medications to stimulate the bowel. This is usually given by the parents at home and professionals will not have to administer it to the child.

The child should never be punished for soiling; it is rarely under his conscious control. On the other hand, he should be rewarded with praise when he successfully uses the toilet. It is a good idea for parents to send along several changes of underwear. When the child soils, he should be assisted in cleaning himself up and changing his clothes. The soiled underwear should be sealed in a plastic bag.

If left untreated, virtually all children will stop soiling at some stage, but will have paid a big price in terms of self-esteem and social isolation. Most children will respond to the treatment regime described, although it may take some months and relapses are not uncommon. Persistence is the key.

When to seek medical advice

Every child with persistent soiling should be checked by a doctor. Usually an X-ray is performed to assess the amount of retention of faeces in the bowel. In addition, the doctor will exclude other rare conditions that may be associated with soiling, like congenital bowel disease or neurological conditions. The doctor will also want to monitor progress and vary the treatment regime as necessary.

Prevention

The chances of developing soiling can be minimised by making sure the child does not become constipated. This is achieved by a well balanced diet, and encouraging the child to go to the toilet immediately when he has an urge, and not hold on. Some children are 'too busy' or engrossed in playing to heed the urge to stool. If they hold on then the urge may pass, and soon this becomes a regular pattern which predisposes them to retention of faeces in the bowel. Early childhood professionals have an important role to play in encouraging or reminding the child to sit on the toilet.

Food allergies

True food allergies are relatively uncommon in young children, though parents will often incorrectly blame food allergy for a host of problems including overactivity and difficult to control behaviour, diarrhoea, rashes, recurrent colds and excess mucus.

Cause

The most common causes of food allergy in young children include peanuts, fish and shellfish, eggs and milk. True food allergy is much less common than the perception held by many parents. Many infants with 'colic' or diarrhoea are wrongly diagnosed as having milk allergy and switched unnecessarily to soy milk. Similarly, a number of parents report improvement in a child's health status when they are taken off dairy foods, even though it is most unlikely that dairy foods were in any way related to the child's perceived problems.

Signs and symptoms

Symptoms vary greatly in severity. In the most severe cases, the child can become suddenly and severely ill (see Allergic reactions page 18). In milder cases, symptoms can include an itchy red rash or hives (see page 89) , tingling of the mouth and tongue, vomiting and diarrhoea.

Treatment

Clearly the most important thing is to avoid the offending food. Children tend to grow out of their allergies as they get older. Where the allergy is so severe that it can cause anaphylactic shock, emergency treatment in the form of an adrenaline injection should always be available. In those rare instances where this is the case, parents will make sure that professionals are fully briefed on what to do.

When to seek medical advice

It is a good idea to have all children who are suspected of having an allergy assessed by a doctor. In many cases the suspicion will be unfounded, and in some instances the allergy can be confirmed by special testing under controlled conditions.

Prevention

The best protection against the development of food allergy is breastfeeding in infancy. Breastfed infants are less likely to develop food allergies. This is especially important when there is a family history of allergies. Then foods should be introduced one at a time, so it will quickly become apparent if there is a problem with a particular food. Where there is a strong family history, a case can be made for delaying the introduction of those foods that are most likely to cause allergy — egg, fish, peanuts, cows' milk — until after 12 months.

There is no evidence that giving infants soy or goats' milk rather than cows' milk protects against the development of food allergy, and these should be avoided.

The role of the early childhood professional in food allergy is critical. Care should be taken not to give the child the offending foods, and they need to take particular care and plan ahead for parties and excursions, so the child who has food allergies can have appropriate food.

Food poisoning

From time to time children may eat something which disagrees with them and results in gastrointestinal symptoms of varying severity. Usually this is the result of food poisoning.

Cause

Food can become contaminated with bacteria in several ways. It may have been inadequately cooked so that bacteria in the food have not been killed. Cooked food that has not been refrigerated allows bacteria to multiply in the higher temperatures. Any food that is prepared in less than hygienic conditions creates the possibility of contamination and resultant food poisoning.

Signs and symptoms

These can include the whole range of gastrointestinal symptoms, such as nausea, vomiting, abdominal pain and diarrhoea. Sometimes more general symptoms such as fever are present as well. The severity depends on the bacteria load, the age of the child and other factors. The symptoms usually begin within a few hours of ingesting the offending food, and last up to 12 hours.

Treatment

Usually food poisoning is self-limited and no specific treatment is needed. Fluids may be offered to the child to maintain hydration. The diarrhoea and vomiting are the body's way of ridding itself of the poison, in this case the contaminated food.

When to seek medical advice

Unless the symptoms are mild and transient, it is wise to seek medical advice so the diagnosis can be confirmed and other causes ruled out.

Prevention

Care always needs to be taken with the handling and preparation of food. The highest standards of hygiene must be maintained.

Gastroenteritis

Gastroenteritis is a common condition in young children. Most are mild and self-limited, but a few are more severe and require active treatment.

Cause

Most cases of gastroenteritis are caused by one of several viruses; bacteria and parasites cause the remainder. The wall of the small intestine becomes inflamed, which disrupts the absorption of intestinal contents, resulting in diarrhoea and sometimes vomiting.

Signs and symptoms

The condition is characterised by the sudden onset of diarrhoea, often accompanied by vomiting and abdominal cramps. The severity varies markedly, from the basically well child with symptoms for a day or two, through to the child with severe persistent diarrhoea and vomiting who becomes rapidly dehydrated and needs urgent treatment. More severe cases may have signs of dehydration (see page 117).

A small number of children, especially the younger ones aged under two years of age, develop lactose (a sugar found in milk) intolerance because of temporary damage to the lining of the bowel wall. Lactose cannot be absorbed, and this leads to a watery, frothy, sweet smelling diarrhoea which can burn the baby's buttocks.

Treatment

Most children have mild gastroenteritis that requires no special treatment other than making sure the child drinks plenty of fluids. More severe cases are treated with oral rehydration fluid. Breast milk should be continued, while if on formula or cows' milk then this can be diluted with water. There is no reason to withhold food if the child is hungry, though bland food should be given during the acute phase. If the child has lactose intolerance then she will need to go onto a special lactose-free formula for a period of time until the lining of the bowel heals and levels of the enzyme lactase are restored.

When to seek medical advice

Most mild cases do not need to be seen by a doctor. If the child is vomiting and unable to keep fluids down, or the diarrhoea is very frequent (more than six bowel movements per day), or the child is showing signs of dehydration (page 117) then medical consultation is advised.

Prevention

Gastroenteritis caused by viruses is very infectious and can spread quickly in child care or other community settings. Spread can be minimised by careful attention to hygiene, such as washing hands and ensuring the cleanliness of toilets and bathrooms. (See also Exclusion Table, page 79.)

Gastro-oesophageal reflux

This is the most common cause of vomiting in children during the first year of life. Mostly it is a nuisance rather than anything serious. It slowly resolves and has usually disappeared completely by the toddler age.

Cause

The valve-like mechanism between the stomach and gullet (oesophagus) does not work properly, thus allowing stomach contents to leak back into the gullet. It slowly begins to work, so that the condition is uncommon after a year of age and rare in toddlers.

Signs and symptoms

Reflux with consequent possetting and small vomits are normal in infants. It is only considered abnormal if large amounts are involved, or it occurs frequently and after each feed. It begins within the first month of birth. The baby vomits large amounts of milk after and in between feeds. In a few infants the vomiting is so severe and persistent that they gain weight poorly, and even lose weight. In some it is thought the acid contents of the stomach may irritate the gullet and cause inflammation and pain. Reflux is thought to be one of the reasons that some babies cry excessively (this is often called 'colic', see page 176), but it is unlikely to be a factor in the vast majority of babies.

Treatment

In most infants reflux is not a serious condition and no treatment is necessary. The main problem seems to be the inconvenience of the baby vomiting over her clothes and the clothes of the parent or carer. As long as the baby is gaining weight and otherwise happy, there is no reason to offer any treatment, knowing that the condition will steadily improve and soon disappear completely.

Simple measures like minimal handling after a feed, and postural measures such as propping her up after feeding, may reduce the amount of vomiting. Some infants benefit from having their feeds thickened. If the reflux is very significant and causing inflammation of the gullet, the infant can be prescribed medicines either to reduce the acidity of the stomach contents, or else reduce the amount of acid secreted into the stomach.

When to seek medical advice

Most infants who vomit a lot, especially if this is associated with poor or erratic weight gain or who appear to be in pain or have inconsolable crying, will need a medical assessment. This is also important to exclude other causes of vomiting.

Hernia

There are two types of herniae in young children. An umbilical hernia and inguinal hernia. The former usually resolves spontaneously, while the latter always need surgery.

Cause

A hernia is a protrusion of a piece of bowel or muscle or other tissue through a gap or weakness in the muscle wall. An inguinal hernia is due to the persistence after birth of a channel between the abdomen and groin.

Signs and symptoms

An inguinal hernia presents as a lump in the groin, usually observed by the parent or caregiver when bathing or changing the child. It is not usually present at birth but can appear any time afterwards and throughout the early years. An umbilical hernia is present from birth and appears as a lump around the belly button. A hernia will easily be able to be reduced (put back into the abdomen) and will always feel hard when the child is crying or coughing. Very rarely, the first presentation of an inguinal hernia is a bowel obstruction with pain and vomiting, and the baby looking pale and sick.

Treatment

An inguinal hernia is always treated surgically, usually within a few days after discovery. If it is left, there is a small but definite chance of strangulation — the piece of bowel becomes 'strangled' by the muscles, resulting in a bowel obstruction. An umbilical hernia usually resolves by the baby's first birthday. Rarely does an umbilical hernia need surgery, unless it is still very large in the toddler years and then mainly for cosmetic reasons. Taping the hernia, or taping it with a coin over it — an old fashioned remedy — does not make it go away any more quickly and the tape may irritate and excoriate the tender skin of the baby. Taping is strongly discouraged.

When to seek medical advice

Any lump in the groin should always be checked immediately by a doctor so that, if it is a hernia, surgery can be arranged without delay.

Nutrition

Malnutrition and other major nutritional problems, apart from obesity, are relatively uncommon in the majority of Australian children, though tragically common amongst Aboriginal Australian children. Nevertheless, establishing the right nutritional patterns from infancy is very important. Here are some principles that can serve as a guide:

▶ Breastfeeding gets the infant off to the best start, and should be encouraged for every mother and every infant.

▶ Where the infant is not breastfed for one reason or another, one of the formulae is used according to the manufacturer's instructions. There are only very minor differences between different brands, and switching from one brand to another should be discouraged.

▶ The main milk source for the first 12 months should be either breastmilk or formula. From about 7–8 months cows' milk can be introduced in small amounts, such as with cereals and in custard.

▶ Solids should not be introduced before 6 months. Breast milk or formula is sufficient for the baby's nutritional needs until then. Crying and irritability in an otherwise healthy infant usually does not mean he is hungry or needs solids to be introduced early.

▶ Milk and food allergies are over-diagnosed. Most babies do perfectly well on breast milk, formula and later cows' milk. They do not need special formulas or soy milk.

▶ Many parents take their child off milk and all dairy foods in the mistaken belief that it causes a range of symptoms in their child, from diarrhoea and poor weight gain through to cough, asthma and excessive mucus. In the vast majority of infants and children this is quite incorrect; dairy products do not contribute to any of these problems.

▶ Most children do not need vitamin supplements provided they are on a reasonable diet. Vitamin deficiencies are rare in Australian children.

▶ Pay attention to the salt and sugar content of food given to the child in the early years. There is some evidence that giving an infant or toddler lots of foods containing sugar gives him a 'sweet tooth' and increases the chances of obesity.

▶ Try to establish good eating habits right from the beginning, making sure the child eats a balanced diet, and choose from each of the food groups. Avoid too much 'junk' food.

Obesity

Obesity is a major and growing public health problem in Australia and other developed countries. Young children who are obese are more likely to continue to be obese as adults, so it is especially important to establish appropriate nutrition and activity patterns at an early age. A child is defined as obese when his weight is more than 120% of the expected weight for his age.

Cause

There are a number of factors that play a role in the development of obesity, including genetic factors, but the main reason simply put is a combination of children eating too much and/or exercising too little. Obesity tends to run in families, and this is likely to be partly genetic and partly environmental. On rare occasions the obesity is caused by a medical or hormonal condition.

There are a number of reasons why obesity is increasing in prevalence so rapidly. There have been major lifestyle changes for families in recent years. A change in eating habits has occurred, with less meal preparation at home and more takeaway foods, which tend to be high in fat. These are called 'energy dense' foods, because they have a lot of calories by weight and serving portion. The change in eating habits has been coupled with a less active and more sedentary lifestyle. These days we have lifts, escalators, the motor car, television (and remote controls so we do not even have to get out of our seat to change the channel) and computer games. Children are far less likely to walk or cycle to school, and to be allowed to play in the street or at the local park.

There is a strong correlation between obesity and the amount of television watched. When children are watching television they are clearly inactive, more likely to be snacking and, in addition, are exposed to a bevy of advertising for various foods, most of which could not be classed as particularly healthy.

Signs and symptoms

Obese children have an altered body shape and in addition to being heavier than other children of the same age may also be taller. In older children and especially adults, obesity is associated with a number of complications, some of which are serious and can be life threatening. However there are also other problems, not least of which is the teasing, poor body image and self-esteem and the effect this has on social relationships.

Treatment

The treatment of established obesity is notoriously difficult at all ages. It is far more effective to prevent obesity or intervene when the children are overweight and on the way to becoming obese. The principle of treatment is to decrease the number of calories consumed while at the same time increasing the number of calories expended. This is easier said than done, for changing the child's and family's eating patterns and activity levels is not easy. The best results are when the whole family participates in the obesity treatment program for the child. Parents monitor and set limits on the amount and type of food eaten by the child, who is encouraged to eat more slowly and discouraged from snacking in between meals. Fatty foods and those with a high sugar content (energy dense foods) are decreased and replaced by more fruit and vegetables and complex carbohydrates such as pasta and rice. The whole family is encouraged to be more conscious of and modify their eating patterns, and to take care with the types of food brought into the house. Sometimes a dietician may help with advice and the selection of a diet appropriate to the age and weight of the child.

Care must be taken with diets in children of any age, but especially in young children, because they are still growing and do need a full range of foods and an optimal level of calories and nutrients. The aim is not to achieve rapid weight loss, but rather to not put weight on. If the weight can be maintained, or reduced very slowly, then the child can 'grow into' his desirable weight.

At the same time, sedentary activities, such as television watching and playing games on the computer, are limited and an increase in activity level planned with the child and family. This only needs to be modest in scope, and the child encouraged to find a range of activities that he enjoys and are therefore more likely to be sustained over the longer term.

Medications and very low calorie diets intended to achieve drastic weight reduction over a short time frame have no place in the treatment of obesity in young children.

When to seek medical advice

If the child is grossly overweight or a medical condition is suspected, then a medical assessment is warranted.

Prevention

Obesity prevention begins in early infancy. Obesity is less common in children who are exclusively breastfed until at least 6 months of age. Solids should not be introduced before 6 months of age. Healthy eating and activity patterns can and should be established in early childhood.

Vomiting

Vomiting is one of the most common symptoms of childhood. There is not a single child who will not vomit from time to time. Mostly these occurrences are of no importance, but occasionally vomiting is an indicator of a serious condition.

Cause

There are many causes of vomiting in infants and young children, and it is regarded as a non-specific symptom rather than indicating a particular condition. Vomiting in infants is usually due to gastro-oesophageal reflux or an infection. In older children it is usually associated with a viral or urinary infection. It can be a manifestation of migraine, or of meningitis or other neurological conditions, or a result of food poisoning or other gastrointestinal condition. Most children will vomit once or twice in association with a minor illness.

Signs and symptoms

If vomiting is persistent and bile stained, it suggests an obstruction to the bowel. Otherwise it is not the vomiting per se but other symptoms and signs the child has that gives clues as to why the child is vomiting. For example, if the vomiting is accompanied by diarrhoea, this suggests gastroenteritis. A cough and runny nose suggests a cold or other viral infection. Vomiting in a young child who has a fever and looks unwell might be due to a urinary tract infection or meningitis.

Treatment

Vomiting itself is never treated in young children. Medicines to stop the vomiting, either by mouth or injection, should never be given to children. They rarely work and can have very unpleasant side effects. It is the underlying condition causing the vomiting that needs to be diagnosed and treated appropriately. Children who are generally unwell due to infection should be given a lighter diet and frequent sips of fluids rather than large meals or large volumes of water which they are more likely to bring back up.

When to seek medical advice

A child who looks unwell with the vomiting should be seen by a doctor as soon as possible. Vomiting that is green or bloodstained, or which is persistent, is always potentially serious and the child needs to be assessed by a doctor.

Worms

Many children suffer from worms. It is of nuisance value rather than a serious condition.

Cause

Pinworms are the most common group to affect children in Australia.

Signs and symptoms

The most common symptom is an itchy anus. The female worms emerge from the anal passage, especially at night, to deposit their eggs. This gives rise to the intense anal itching, especially at night, which suggests that worms might be the cause. Infection in more than one family member is common. The eggs can survive on bedding or clothes for up to two weeks, and re-infection is common.

Treatment

Worms are easily and successfully treated by medicine or tablets taken by mouth as a single dose, though a second dose two weeks later is usually recommended. The child's bedclothes and pyjamas should be washed in hot water and his fingernails cut short and hands washed carefully after going to the toilet.

Neurological

Convulsions

Convulsions, sometimes called seizures or fits, are sudden transient changes in consciousness and motor tone.

Cause

Convulsions are caused by abnormal electrical impulses in the brain; these can be due to a number of causes. In young children the commonest cause is fever. About 3–4% of children under the age of 5 years will have a febrile seizure, associated with a fever. For reasons that are unclear, the rapid rise in the body temperature causes abnormal electrical discharges which results in the convulsion. Most have a single episode.

Recurrent convulsions are called epilepsy. Sometimes there is scarring of part of the brain that is then responsible for the abnormal electrical discharges. The scarring can be due to cerebral palsy (see page 174), or a head injury. In most children with epilepsy no specific cause can be found, but the electrical waves in the brain are persistently abnormal.

Signs and symptoms

There are different types of epilepsy, with different clinical features. The most common type of seizure is called grand mal and this is the clinical type also seen in a febrile convulsion. It is characterised by sudden stiffening of the body, followed by uncontrollable jerking movements which last anywhere from seconds to a few minutes, thought it may seem longer. The child's eyes roll to the back of his head, and the mouth and teeth are clenched. Sometimes there may be frothing of the mouth, and often there is loss of control of bladder and bowels. The child may fall to the ground or slump in his chair. Following the convulsion the child will usually be very drowsy and will sleep for an hour or so.

Other forms of epilepsy are characterised by different clinical features. In some types only certain parts of the body are involved and there is no loss of consciousness. In another form, called petit mal epilepsy, the child simply stares for a few seconds (called an *absence*), and then continues with what he was doing as if nothing has happened.

A febrile seizure, the most common in young children, lasts for no longer that five minutes and often much less. The child may be drowsy afterwards, but makes a full recovery. About one in four children will have more than one febrile convulsion. They are always associated with a fever, usually caused by a virus or an ear infection. Sometimes the onset of the fever is so rapid that the convulsion occurs before there are other signs indicating that the child has an infection and is unwell. There are no long-term effects of febrile seizures; in particular they do not cause brain damage or future learning difficulties.

Treatment

Observing a child who is fitting is very scary for professionals involved with children, but especially for parents. Parents whose children have had a convulsion report that they thought the child was going to die. The first and most important aspect of management of the convulsion is to stay as calm as possible. Lay the child on the ground with his head turned to one side, and follow instructions in the emergencies section under convulsions (page 26). The convulsion lasts only a few minutes and usually stops before any treatment can be given. The most important aspect of treatment is to keep the child safe and prevent him from hurting himself.

Children with epilepsy will always be taking one or more medications. The aim of treatment is to prevent seizures from recurring or, if that is not possible, then minimising their frequency and severity. Many children with epilepsy will completely 'grow out' of the condition over time, while in others they are greatly reduced as they get older.

Febrile seizures occur once only in most children. Many parents and professionals are anxious about the child having another convulsion every time he gets a fever. While this is understandable, it is an anxiety unfounded for most children. It is reasonable to give the child paracetamol whenever he has a fever, although many febrile seizures seem to occur in the very early stage of an illness when the fever is rapidly rising and before the illness is evident.

When to seek medical advice

Children with epilepsy will be under the care of a doctor, usually a specialist such as a paediatrician or paediatric neurologist. They will review the child regularly and finetune the medications in order to prevent or minimise the number of convulsions.

Any child who has a first convulsion should be seen as soon as possible by a doctor, who will organise tests including recording the brain's electrical activity with an EEG (electroencephalogram). If the convulsion was associated with a fever, the child should be seen immediately to find the source of the fever, and make sure that it is nothing serious like meningitis.

Prevention

Children with epilepsy who are on medications already will have the dose and blood levels closely monitored by their doctor to make sure that they are appropriate and offer the best chance of preventing further seizures. A few children with recurrent febrile seizures may also be prescribed anticonvulsant medication to prevent further seizures from occurring.

Deafness (hearing loss)

The severity of deafness in young children varies greatly, from those who have a severe and permanent hearing loss from birth (sensorineural) to those who have a temporary hearing loss associated with an ear infection (conductive).

Adequate hearing is essential for normal language development and so hearing loss, depending on its type, severity and duration, places the child at risk of speech and language problems.

Sensorineural hearing loss

Cause

This type of hearing loss is due to abnormal function of part of the inner ear or part of the brain concerned with hearing. It is usually congenital (present from birth), though may be acquired later as the result of meningitis or head injury or the side effects of certain groups of drugs. Some forms of deafness are genetically inherited and run in families.

Signs and symptoms

The newborn infant may be suspected of having a hearing loss because she has one of the 'risk factors' for deafness (see table, page 139). The parents may notice that their baby does not startle at loud noises or respond to their voice, and later will not turn to sound, and after six months engage in less babbling and vocalisation than expected. **A child is never too young to have a hearing test.** She can be tested shortly after birth before she leaves the hospital — this is the goal for those babies that have one of the major risk factors, but soon there will be programs across Australia where all babies will have their hearing tested in the hospital or shortly after discharge.

Treatment

The earlier the deafness is diagnosed and treated the better. Most children with moderate to severe deafness will need a hearing aid, and the aim is to try to fit this earlier than 6 months to give the child the best possible chance of optimal speech and language development. The fitting of a hearing aid is a specialised process that is performed free of charge in Australia by Australian Hearing Services, and the parents and family also undergo an intense educational and support program to teach them how to communicate with a deaf child and promote optimal language development. Some children may be suitable for a cochlear implant, which is able to restore hearing almost to normal levels in carefully selected patients.

When to seek medical advice

If parents or early childhood professionals suspect that the infant or child may have difficulty hearing, then medical advice should be sought immediately, and the child referred to an audiologist for a formal hearing test.

Prevention

Some of the causes of sensorineural deafness, such as maternal rubella during pregnancy, can be theoretically prevented.

Conductive hearing loss

Cause

This is associated with an ear infection (page 46). Most ear infections will cause a variable loss of hearing in the affected ear, and as the infection resolves the hearing returns to normal. However, some children have a persistent hearing loss due to recurrent ear infections which lead to chronic otitis media or glue ear (see page 46).

Signs and symptoms

The clinical features of ear infections can be found on page 46. Children with recurrent ear infections may continue to have symptoms each time. However many children with developing conductive hearing loss may not have symptoms of infection at all. There may be suspicion of hearing loss because of delayed language, or else because the child may seem hard of hearing. She may not follow instructions or ask to have them repeated, or speak loudly or have the television always turned right up.

Treatment

This depends on the child, the severity and duration of the condition, and her age. Most children will initially be treated with several courses of antibiotics, and some will take them for several months, perhaps right throughout the winter. Some children may go on to surgery to suck out the fluid, and some will have grommets or ventilating tubes placed in their ears to drain the fluid responsible for the hearing loss. Children with conductive hearing loss rarely need to have a hearing aid fitted.

When to seek medical advice

Children with ear infections should be seen by a doctor each time they occur. If there is suspicion that the child may have difficulty hearing, then early referral for a hearing test and medical assessment is essential. Do not wait. Children about whom there is a concern about their hearing must have a formal hearing test performed as soon as possible. Professionals who are worried that a child may not be hearing properly should share this concern with the parents, who should be advised to organise a formal hearing test as soon as possible.

The child at risk for hearing loss

Children who have one or more of these risk factors have a higher chance of having a hearing loss (though this does not mean that they *will* have one).

Babies	Parental concern about hearing
	Family history of deafness or hearing loss
	Maternal infection during pregnancy with rubella, CMV, toxoplasmosis
	Severe jaundice
	Congenital abnormalities of the head and neck
	Birthweight less than 1500 grams, needed antibiotics while in hospital, or in intensive care for more than 3 days after birth
	Meningitis
	Repeated ear infections
Toddlers and older children	Concern about hearing held by parent or professional
	Recurrent ear infections
	Delayed language or speech, or developmental delay
	Meningitis
	Problems with attention, concentration, or easy distraction
	Wanting to have things repeated, not following instructions or directions, speaking in loud voice, having television loud

If parents or professionals have a concern about hearing at any age, the child should be referred immediately for a formal hearing test to an audiologist or paediatric specialist. The child is never too young for a hearing test.

Dizziness

Some children may complain of feeling dizzy. They know what this feels like when they spin around and around during play, but otherwise it is an unusual symptom that children rarely complain about. Some viral infections may be associated with dizziness, and an ear infection may distort the child's balance. If the child says he feels dizzy, or if he seems unsteady when walking or standing, it is best to have him checked by a doctor.

Headache

Headache is a common complaint in children of all ages, though the younger the child the more difficulty she will have in being able to localise the pain and being able to articulate it.

Cause

The commonest cause of headache in young children is that associated with viral infections, such as a cold or influenza. They can also be caused by migraine (see page 143), anxiety or stress, and eye strain. Rarely it can be a manifestation of something more serious, such as meningitis or a brain tumour, though in these conditions headache is but one of a number of pointers to the underlying condition.

Signs and symptoms

The symptoms vary according to the cause. Young children will not be able to describe the nature of the pain, whether it is sharp or dull, throbbing or constant. They may be able to localise it to some extent, but they are much more likely simply to say that their head hurts. Sometimes they may complain that the light hurts their eyes. There will be other features of the condition that has caused the headache — fever, sore throat or ear, runny nose.

Treatment

It is best to let the child dictate the level of treatment. If she is happy going on playing, then there is no need to do anything. On the other hand if the headache causes her to lose interest in her usual activities, it helps to keep her quiet, perhaps have her lie down, and if the pain and discomfort does not go away in half an hour then to give paracetamol in the appropriate dose.

When to seek medical advice

If the headache persists despite the simple measures outlined above, or if it recurs frequently, then the child should be seen by a doctor. If the headache is associated with drowsiness or confusion, if she complains of light hurting her eyes, is unsteady walking, or looks sick, then immediate medical attention is advised.

Meningitis

Meningitis is an infection of the meninges, the delicate membrane which covers the brain and spinal cord. It is a serious and potentially life threatening condition that can have major and permanent consequences. It is less common than it used to be because of new vaccines given to children that protect against several of the bacteria that cause meningitis.

Cause

Meningitis in young children can be caused by a variety of viruses and bacteria. There are now vaccines against the three common bacteria that cause meningitis — haemophilus influenzae, pneumococcus and meningococcus — so it is seen less commonly these days. (This is another reason to make sure your child is fully immunised. Information about immunisation, including the current schedule, can be found at <**http://immunise.health.gov.au**>.

Signs and symptoms

Meningitis often follows what appears to be a simple cold or upper respiratory infection. The classic symptoms are headache, stiff neck, aversion to light, and nausea and vomiting. However in young children these symptoms are not as clear, and the child just looks pale and unwell, with a high fever, listless and irritable, and sometimes drowsy. Meningitis is a medical emergency, and urgent medical attention is essential if it is suspected.

Treatment

If meningitis is suspected, the child is taken to hospital for assessment, which includes a lumbar puncture. This procedure consists of a needle being inserted into the child's spinal canal and a few drops of spinal fluid checked to see if it contains cells and other signs of infection. Where bacterial meningitis is confirmed, the child is admitted to hospital for a week or longer, and antibiotics given intravenously. If the meningitis is due to a virus, the child may still be admitted depending on how sick he is, but antibiotics are not necessary and the child is usually discharged earlier.

When to seek medical advice

If there are symptoms and signs suggesting even a remote possibility of meningitis, the child should be seen by a doctor as a matter of urgency.

Prevention

Making sure that all children are fully immunised is the best way to prevent meningitis.

Migraine

Migraine is not common in young children, and its prevalence increases as children get older.

Cause

The cause of migraine is uncertain. It tends to run in families, so clearly has a genetic component. Sometimes a trigger factor can be identified, such as stress or a certain type of food.

Signs and symptoms

Children do not have the classic features of migraine seen in adults. Abdominal symptoms such as nausea, abdominal pain and vomiting are prominent in children, and the headache may not be a major feature. The child looks pale and may be sweaty. The migraine may last a few hours and be followed by sleep. During an attack the child will want to lie down, and will complain of glare and of light hurting his eyes.

Treatment

During an attack the child will prefer to lie quietly in a darkened room, and will probably not feel like eating or drinking. Paracetamol given early in an attack will likely make a difference and may even ward off some of the symptoms. An attempt is made to identify and avoid trigger factors. If the child is getting very frequent attacks of migraine, medicines given on a daily basis to try to prevent the attacks may be considered; these should only be prescribed by a specialist following a complete assessment.

When to seek medical advice

Any child with more than the occasional headache should be seen by a doctor.

Prevention

If trigger factors can be identified, they should be avoided wherever possible.

Muscles and bones

Arthritis

This is relatively uncommon in young children, but when present and severe can significantly limit the child's functioning and physical mobility.

Cause

The causes of arthritis include a juvenile version of rheumatoid arthritis, infections (septic arthritis, post infectious arthritis) and non-specific causes such as irritable hip.

Signs and symptoms

These vary according to the cause, and can range from acute and transient arthritis through to chronic arthritis that persists throughout childhood. The child complains of varying degrees of pain and limited movement in one or more joints, which may be reddened, swollen, hot to touch and tender. Depending on the cause, there may be other signs also, such as a rash or fever.

Treatment

This depends on the cause. For acute conditions it can include rest, pain relief and anti-inflammatory medications. More severe and chronic conditions require ongoing specialist treatment, and a number of medications including steroids and, sometimes, weekly injections are prescribed. In an early childhood setting, the child might have reduced mobility or reduced tolerance of physical activity.

When to seek medical advice

Any child who complains of pain or soreness of one or more joints should be seen by a doctor so that a diagnosis can be made and appropriate treatment implemented as necessary.

Bruises

Many young children will have bruises from time to time, on their legs and arms in particular. These are usually of no consequence and part of the rough and tumble of childhood, but very occasionally they may be a manifestation of something serious.

Cause

Bruises are caused by bleeding into the skin from small blood vessels which have burst, almost always in response to trauma of some kind. Mostly this is quite a normal and inevitable part of growing up, especially in boys. Rarely there is an underlying bleeding or clotting disorder, either inherited or as the result of a specific condition such as an infection or leukaemia. Children who have been physically abused can also present with bruising.

Signs and symptoms

The bruising is most often seen on the legs (especially the shins) and arms. There will usually be a number of small bruises in varying stages of resolution. As they resolve, they change colour from the original dark almost black colour to various hues of blue and brown and yellow until they disappear completely. Child abuse is suspected when the bruising is on the trunk, the buttocks and back in particular, or the face (see Child abuse, page 203). If the bruising is due to an underlying bleeding or clotting disorder, there will be a history of easy bruising and bleeding from birth, or other manifestations that will provide clues that this is a departure from normal.

Treatment

No active treatment of bruising is necessary in most cases. Where a child falls over and knocks himself, an ice pack, that is first wrapped in a tea towel or cloth, applied immediately and left on for 15 minutes may reduce the amount of bruising.

When to seek medical advice

It is hard to specify how much bruising can be considered to be 'normal' in a young child. He should be seen by a doctor if a parent or early childhood professional considers that the bruising is excessive, or if there is easy associated bleeding, for example from the nose, or if there are other features suggesting either the possibility of child abuse or an underlying medical condition.

Fractures

Bones of young children can be easily broken by falls or collisions, but they also heal very quickly. Broken bones in children heal at a much faster rate than adults. Sometimes it is apparent that the child has suffered a fractured or broken bone; this is due to deformity, with parts of the limb at the wrong angle to each other, or the degree of severe pain and swelling, and/or reluctance to move the affected body part.

However, the definitive diagnosis of a fracture can only be made by X-ray and this should be organised as soon as possible. Until the child can be seen by a doctor or taken to hospital, the principles of management are to relieve pain, keep the child as comfortable as possible, and try to avoid moving the limb or body part that is broken. A splint can be made with a piece of wood and a bandage or torn up strip of material, and this is effective in immobilising the limb (see Fractures and dislocations, page 30).

Growing pains

This is a term used to describe pains in the legs and joints that occur commonly in childhood. It is especially common in school-age children, but can also be seen at a younger age.

Cause

The cause of growing pains is not known, but it is most unlikely that it has anything to do with the growth of the child or the bones or muscles, so in this sense it is a misnomer. In many children it is associated with abdominal pain and headaches, suggesting it may be a response to stress. Some children with growing pains have a temperament profile that suggests these children are more intense and have a lower threshold of sensitivity.

Signs and symptoms

The child complains of an ache or burning sensation in the legs — the feet, calves, thighs or joints. The pain can also occur in the arms, though this is less common. The pain is often especially persistent during the night, when it may wake the child from sleep, but can occur during the daytime as well. Growing pains tend to come and go, rather than being present all the time, and they tend to improve and then disappear as the child gets older. They are rarely severe enough to interfere with daily activities, and are not present when she is active and running around. The child remains otherwise well.

Treatment

There is no specific treatment, and often all that is needed is to reassure the child. Some children seem to respond to heat, and others to massage, and occasionally paracetamol can be given. There is no need to restrict activity.

When to seek medical advice

If the pains are severe and persistent, or if there are other features such as a limp or fever or the child looks unwell, then medical assessment is advised.

Limp

This is relatively common in childhood. Mostly it is not serious and the child is quickly back to normal, but occasionally it heralds a more serious condition.

Cause

There are a number of causes of limp. Acute onset of limp in a young child may be due to trauma — a fracture or bruise, or an infection of the bone or one of the joints of the leg, most commonly the hip. Limp that has been present for some time may indicate arthritis, cerebral palsy (page 174), congenital dislocation of the hip, or a developmental defect of the hip joint.

Signs and symptoms

The child favours his good leg, and puts as little weight as possible on the affected leg. The young child will have difficulty localising or describing the pain. Sometimes there are other features that will point to the cause, such as a history of recent trauma. Fever, loss of appetite and irritability indicate a possible infection. Examination of the child may show limited movement of one of his legs, and pain in a joint when further active movement is attempted.

Treatment

This depends on the cause. In many children the limp will go away after a few hours or a day or two, and rest is all that is needed. Once the diagnosis is established — often requiring blood tests and special X-rays — then treatment specific to the condition is instituted.

When to seek medical advice

Any child who limps for more than a few hours, especially if he looks unwell or has a fever, should be seen by a doctor as soon as possible.

Orthopaedic problems

Young children commonly have a number of orthopaedic problems that give concern to parents, though most are not of serious concern.

Bow legs

This refers to the outward bowing of the legs; when the child stands with feet together, the ankles touch but the knees are several centimetres apart. This is normal, and is seen especially in the first three or four years of life. It tends to improve as the child grows older. No treatment is needed.

Dislocated hip

This is commonly called congenital dislocation of the hip (CDH) meaning that the hip is dislocated from birth, or developmental dysplasia of the hip (DDH). The hip joint is a ball and socket joint. In DDH the top of the thighbone (the ball) does not sit properly in the socket of the hip bone. It is more common in girls, and is usually only one side, though about a quarter occur on both sides. It is more common in breech births because of the position of the legs in the womb during pregnancy. If it is detected during infancy, soon after birth, then treatment is straightforward. The child wears a special harness or splint for about three months. This keeps the legs apart and ensures that the hip joint is in its proper place until the capsule of the joint strengthens and matures. The child's hip joint then develops normally. However, when the diagnosis is delayed, treatment is much more complex and surgery is almost always needed. DDH is one of the possible causes of limp in young children.

Flat feet

All infants have flat feet due to the fat that fills in the spaces between the bones and the ligaments of the sole of the feet. Once children begin to walk the arch of the foot becomes more defined, and most children of school age no longer have flat feet. In the small number of children who do not develop an arch and therefore continue to have flat feet, no treatment is necessary or effective. In particular special 'orthopaedic' shoes or inserts are not effective. If the child's feet hurt when walking or running, then specialist referral is indicated; however this is most unusual.

Knock knees

This is the opposite of bow legs. When the child stands with his feet together, his knees are touching, but there is a space between his ankles. Like bow legs, this is normally seen in young children, becoming most obvious in the toddler period and persisting up until about eight years of age. No treatment is indicated.

Pigeon toes

Babies and toddlers will often have their feet pointing inwards. This is due to the alignment of the hip, leg or thigh bones, which corrects itself as the child grows older. Occasionally it is due to the alignment of the bones in the foot itself. If it is still present at school age then the child should be seen by a paediatric orthopaedic surgeon.

Diabetes

Diabetes is one of the more common chronic medical conditions of childhood, though it is not that common in the preschool period.

Cause

Diabetes is due to a failure of insulin production by the pancreas. Insulin is an essential body hormone which is involved in the metabolism of glucose. Without insulin, glucose accumulates in the blood stream rather than entering the cells where it is normally metabolised to produce energy.

Signs and symptoms

The onset of diabetes is over several weeks. The child is increasingly thirsty, drinking great volumes of fluids and passing large quantities of urine. This leads to an increased frequency of urination and sometimes to bedwetting. There is often a gradual loss of weight, and he may become tired with little energy and be irritable. There may be nausea and sometimes vomiting, and occasionally the child may present in diabetic coma.

Treatment

The child is admitted to hospital initially where the diagnosis is confirmed and a management regime implemented. This consists of insulin injections once or twice a day, a strictly controlled diet, and regular testing of blood and urine to adjust the insulin dosage. Older children are taught to manage the condition themselves, with supervision from their parents. However in the young child it is the parent who must check the blood, supervise the diet and give the insulin injections.

Implications for early childhood professionals

The child with diabetes is indistinguishable from his peers in terms of day-to-day activities. In the early childhood setting he needs no special treatment, except to be aware of when his sugar levels in the blood are dropping. This is referred to as hypoglycaemia, or 'having a hypo'. This is due to an imbalance between the levels of insulin and the level of glucose circulating in his bloodstream. The treatment of a hypo is to be given glucose by mouth, in the form of a drink or something to eat. Early childhood professionals who have a child with diabetes in their care will need to talk to his parents to ensure they understand the symptoms and know what to do.

Normal development and behaviour
Brain development

Research in recent years has given us a new understanding of brain development in infants and young children. This development begins in the uterus before birth and continues throughout childhood.

This research reinforces the importance of good nutrition during pregnancy, along with the avoidance of smoking, and avoiding or minimising alcohol ingestion. Regular antenatal care is important so that any problems or potential problems, such as issues to do with maternal health, can be identified early.

But it is the new knowledge about how the brain develops after birth that is especially important. We now know that infants are born with many billions of brain cells connected by a complex system of wiring (called synapses) and support structures. Information flow between the brain cells and the different parts of the brain and between the brain and nerve cells in other parts of the body flow through these connections. This information flow is responsible for motor, sensory, cognitive and emotional development — how we move, see, hear, think, act and feel.

The stimuli and experiences the infant receives as a result of interacting with her caregivers — parents, extended family, early childhood professionals, and others in her immediate environment — have a direct influence on how these connections develop. Children learn within the context of relationships. The quality of those relationships, and indeed of the whole caretaking environment, is crucially important, along with genetic and biological factors, in shaping the architecture of the developing brain. This in turn has long-term implications for the way the child develops and behaves later in life. There is some evidence that difficulties with self-regulation behaviours — attentional problems, aggression, and social difficulties — may have their origins in the early years of life.

On the other hand there is accumulating research evidence that a stimulating and nurturing environment, along with protection from disease and good nutrition, beginning with breastfeeding, can improve outcomes in a range of domains in children who for one reason or another are at risk of having later problems. Reading regularly to children from an early age, as young as six months, has been shown not only to improve language skills but decrease the chance of them having literacy problems when they begin formal schooling.

This is not about making children smarter, or having them read earlier. It is about taking note of the evidence that the early years of life are critically important in setting the foundations for the whole of the life cycle. Getting the child off to a good start by providing a nurturing, safe, stimulating and consistent environment is the aim of all families and early childhood professionals. There is disturbing evidence that many problems much later in life, including criminality, mental health problems, school and reading difficulties, and medical conditions such as obesity and diabetes, can often be traced back to pathways that begin in the early years of life.

This is why academics, researchers and other professionals advocate high standards in child care and family day care, as well as any setting which looks after or teaches young children. The research points to the need for high quality child care with appropriate staffing ratios and caring and well trained staff. Similar considerations apply to other early childhood settings such as preschools. This does not mean that if a child does not have the benefit of a good caretaking environment she will invariably have later problems. Nor does it mean that it is all over by three years of age. It simply means that those early years are important, not just now but for the child's future as well.

Detailed descriptions of some of this research can be found on a website specially developed for early childhood professionals. The web address is <**http://www.ecconnections.com.au**>. There are also links to other useful early childhood websites.

Language and speech development

Language is an innate ability in humans, and will develop invariably provided the child has normal hearing, the anatomy of the mouth, palate and tongue is intact, and appropriate stimulation is received from parents, caregivers and other children. Communication and language develops along a predictable sequence, though of course there is considerable variability between children. Infants babble from about 6 months, and then begin to make repetitive sound such as da-da-da or ma-ma-ma. Young children will listen attentively to sounds made by parents and caregivers. This can be simply adults talking to the child, or singing, or repeating the babble back to him. This sort of stimulation is very important in facilitating the development of language. Young children who have the benefit of a rich language environment are likely to do better in attainment of language skills than those who are reared in a language poor environment.

Sometime between 6 and 12 months the child may begin to imitate speech sounds, and soon after that say simple words like mama and dada with meaning. In the second and third years of life there is a virtual explosion of language, with a rapidly emerging vocabulary and increased comprehension of instructions and commands and language spoken by parents and caregivers. Toddlers begin to string words together, initially two at a time and then phrases and sentences.

Both speech and comprehension depend on adequate hearing. If the child has a hearing loss, partial or total, permanent or fluctuating, then language may be absent or delayed, or there may be problems of articulation or intelligibility.

The rate of language development depends on a number of factors. Girls tend to be more advanced than boys in their language development. Second and later born children may either be faster in developing language (because they have siblings to stimulate and speak to them) or slower (because their siblings learn to understand their non-verbal communication and translate the these needs to parents without the need for language). The temperament of a child (see page 159) may also be a factor. A shy, inhibited child may tend to hold back in communication, whereas the opposite may be true for an outgoing, confident child.

Normal development and developmental milestones

Although no two children follow exactly the same path in their development, there is remarkable consistency in development given its complexity and all the biological and environmental variables that influence it. One only has to think of the newborn infant on the one hand, and the 5-year-old beginning school on the other, to have a sense of how astounding this developmental progression really is.

Below is a list of common milestones and the ages that children reach them. Remember there is a great deal of individual variability between children, so this should be taken as a guide only. *Nevertheless, if there is any doubt about a child's development, then an early assessment by a paediatrician or other specialist should be organised as soon as possible.*

Developmental milestone	Average age
Social smile	6 weeks
Follows with eyes past midline	6 weeks
Laughs	8–12 weeks
Turns to voice	4 months
Sits with support	4–6 months
Sits without support	6–9 months
Feeds self biscuit	6–8 months
Babbles	6–9 months
Crawls	6–9 months
Mama/dada (no meaning)	8–9 months
Mama/dada (with meaning)	10–18 months
Understands several words	12–15 months
Waves goodbye	8–12 months
Stands holding on	6–10 months
Walks holding on	8–12 months
Plays peek-a boo	9–10 months
Walks alone	10–15 months
Speaks single words	12–16 months
Points to body parts	14–24 months
Combines two words	15–24 months
Climbs stairs	15–20 months
Uses spoon	15–24 months
Helps with clothing	18–26 months
Jumps in place	20–30 months
Rides tricycle	24–36 months
Bowel control	2–4 years
Bladder control	2–4 years

School readiness

Beginning school is a major transition in the life of the child, as well as his family. The first year is important in setting the stage for learning, for shaping attitudes to school and motivation for learning, and for the development of social relationships and self-esteem. It is important not to send the child to school before he is ready, and yet establishing whether he is ready can sometimes be difficult.

School readiness is usually defined by chronological age. In Australia, there are differences in school starting age from state to state, with the range spanning 4½ to 5½ years. Most states have an enrolment only at the beginning of the school year, some have several enrolments during the year, and some allow continuous enrolment so the child begins school at the time he reaches a certain age. While it is not unreasonable from a logistic and organisational point of view to make age the criterion for beginning school, and this seems to work for most children, there is a good deal of variability in development and maturation at this age. This means that most children are ready for school at round about five years of age, but some are not.

How can we be sure a child is ready to begin school? This is a question that is not easily answered. There are a number of factors, apart from age, that need to be taken into account. The child needs to be physically ready and sturdy enough to cope with school. He needs to be independent so he can attend to his toilet needs, and be able to dress and undress without help. He needs to be able to socialise with his peers, and be able to concentrate and stay focused on tasks that a formal learning situation demands. He needs to be emotionally mature enough to be left all day away from his parents, and he needs to have the language and other developmental skills to be able to begin formal learning.

Family and local community factors also need to be taken into account. Some states only offer a single year of kindergarten, so unless the child is delayed developmentally or the parents choose a private preschool, a second year is not an option. Some families may decide on school because of financial reasons, with both parents needing to work.

There is no single test that can reliably provide the answer as to whether the child is ready for school. The considered opinion of an experienced kindergarten teacher is often said to be as reliable as any test, because of the experience she has had and the fact that she is likely to take into account a myriad of factors that are impossible to put into a readiness test. Maturation in the preschool age is uneven, with great variability in rates of development. For example, a child may be perceived as not ready in October but ready by the beginning of the school year only a few months later. It is therefore very important to adopt a flexible attitude to the timing of school entry for a particular child.

Sleep

Although there is considerable variability in individual sleep patterns and requirements, all children do go through fairly predictable cycles of sleep.

Newborn

The newborn infant sleeps for up to 20 hours out of 24, usually in spells of two to four hours at a time. She will wake only when she is hungry or uncomfortable. In the first few weeks following the birth, the patterns may be unpredictable, and it may take some time for her to settle down into any sort of routine.

Infant

By 6 weeks of age, infants are awake for longer periods during the day, as they take an increased interest in their surroundings and begin to interact more with the mother or caregiver. By 6 months, rather than sleeping most of the time, they are awake and playing or interacting for longer periods, and have several naps during the day. Some may already be sleeping most of the night.

Between 6 and 12 months, there continues to be considerable change in sleeping patterns. Most infants will be sleeping for 10–12 hours during the night. Some will sleep all night, whereas others may wake once or twice but readily go back to sleep. This is also the time when dysfunctional sleep patterns also begin, with some infants either not getting into a predictable sleep pattern, or getting into patterns that cause their parents problems, for example waking through the night and being difficult to settle.

Toddler

Toddlers' sleep patterns tend to be geared to household routines. They are awake for long periods, having a nap in the afternoon, or perhaps still two naps a day. This depends somewhat on the routines of the family or the early childhood centre. Most will sleep all night, though many parents will present with problems of night waking or of difficulties getting the child to bed at night time. This is the commonest time for children to be reported as having sleep problems. Sometimes this is one of a number of behaviours that cause parents concern. At other times it is a specific problem of sleep that causes difficulties (see Sleep problems, page 188).

Preschool

Most preschoolers sleep all night, usually for 10–12 hours. Some will nap during the day, depending a lot on family routines, but others will not need to sleep during the day.

Teeth

Children get their first teeth between 6 and 9 months of age, and from then teeth erupt regularly. A good rule of thumb to predict the number of teeth is to calculate seven plus one month for each tooth. For example a child of twelve months would be expected to have five or six teeth. By the age of three years, children will have their full complement of twenty primary or milk teeth.

Children who are teething can become irritable, drool excessively and have their sleep affected. This is due to the soreness and sometimes inflammation as the teeth push up through the gum. The discomfort can be eased by giving the child a rusk or teething ring to chew on. Young children who are teething will often chew on things they put in their mouth, and this is a good indication that they are having some discomfort from teething. The pressure of these objects against the gum is soothing. Sometimes if the child is especially irritable or having disturbed sleep, paracetamol can be given.

Contrary to popular opinion, teething does *not* cause fever, diarrhoea, ear infections, or other ailments. All of these are common in young children, who also are at the age where they happen to be teething, and so they are wrongly linked together.

Fluoridation has greatly reduced the incidence of tooth decay in children. Many communities have their water fluoridated; where this is not the case, then fluoride supplements should be given to the child. There are other things apart from fluoridation that parents and professionals can do to ensure that children have healthy teeth. Young children should never be allowed to go to bed with a bottle in their mouth. This will almost inevitably cause dental caries. Bottles should be used for feeding, not pacifying. Sweet substances, such as honey or jam, should never be smeared on a dummy. Once the child is old enough to rinse and spit, encourage him to get into the routine of regular tooth brushing. Parents or caregivers can brush the teeth of younger children.

Temperament

In times gone by, it was commonly thought that all children were much the same in terms of the way they reacted to the outside world. We now understand that there are major individual differences amongst children, and often these differences are noticeable from soon after birth. Temperament is used to describe these individual differences. Temperament is genetic in origin, though it is continually being modified by the child's experience of the environment.

A child's temperament has been described as a sort of filter through which she experiences and interacts with the environment. It is the behavioural style of the child, and can be measured using a series of parent-completed questionnaires. Temperament can be categorised into *difficult, easy*, and *slow to warm up* temperament types. Children with a *difficult* temperament are much more likely to be difficult for parents and professionals alike. As infants they are more likely to have excessive crying and 'colic'; and to have sleep problems. As toddlers, they are more likely to have difficult behaviours such as temper tantrums, sleep problems, and aggressive behaviour.

On the other hand those with an *easy* temperament are more likely to be easy to manage, while those who have a *slow to warm up* temperament are likely to adapt slowly to new situations as they take time to get used to things, are often held back and shy, and may be initially difficult until they have had time to adjust.

Parents and caregivers need to be aware of the temperament of the child, and try to adjust the way they interact with the child accordingly. Flexibility is the key. Know that different children may react differently to the same situation. What works well for one child may not be so successful for others. For example, a slow to warm up child will not readily take to changes in routines or new situations. She may hand tightly onto a parent or caregiver, exhibiting great reluctance for example to engage in play situations or interact with her peers. There is no point pushing her, for this will likely make matters worse. An appreciation that this child has a different temperament type and needs different handling will allow a gentle and unhurried approach which will in time see the child slowly adapting and joining in.

The best outcomes for children are realised when it is appreciated that the one approach does not suit all children. The child rearing style of parents and style of teaching needs to be modified to make sure there is a good fit with each child's temperament characteristics. It follows then that there is no single way to approach children, whether it be feeding, toilet-training, discipline, teaching, or any other area of functioning. Each child must be treated as an individual.

Problems of development and behaviour

Aggressive behaviour

Aggressive behaviour in children is one of the most difficult of all behaviours to manage. Unfortunately it is one of the most stable of the behaviour problems in childhood, so aggressive youngsters have a good chance of continuing their aggressive behaviour as they reach school age and beyond. It most commonly begins in the toddler period, and while for many children is a transient developmental phase that does not last, for others it becomes more of a problem over time.

Cause

It is likely that the causes of aggression are multifactorial. It is much more common in boys, and tends to run in families. It is difficult to know to what extent this may be inherited and to what extent it is the result of social learning. If a child grows up in a family environment where there is poor and inconsistent limit setting and verbal and physical aggression is common, he will learn that this is a reasonable way to settle arguments or to display his own anger or frustration. Children with an active, outgoing temperament are more likely than shy children to display aggressive, boisterous behaviour. In some families, aggression is encouraged, especially in boys. Parents boast that their son is 'tough', and aggression is openly admired and encouraged in many forms of sport. There is also concern about the exposure of young children to violence on TV and video games, with mounting evidence that this may contribute to a culture where aggression is seen as an acceptable and even desirable form of behaviour.

Signs and symptoms

Occasional bursts of aggression are not uncommon in young children, and it is often difficult to draw the distinction between the rough and tumble of normal play and inappropriately aggressive or violent behaviour. Often it begins around the issue of sharing toys and playing with peers. Some children become angry when frustrated or provoked, and lash out verbally or physically. Usually they can be distracted or consoled, so the episode is quickly over and occurs infrequently.

However, a small number of children seem to display this behaviour frequently, and it may get worse with time. Often it is unpredictable and there seems little apparent reason for aggressive outbursts. If severe and persistent, there are usually social and often emotional consequences for the child. He will likely become socially isolated and have difficulty making and keeping friends, with an inevitable effect on his self-esteem.

Parents may report that the child is aggressive at home, but does not seem to be so in the early childhood setting. This suggests poor or inconsistent limit setting by the parents at home, or that the behaviour is being unwittingly reinforced by the parents' reaction to it.

Management

Like most other behavioural problems, aggressive behaviour is best managed at an early stage, before it becomes entrenched and then much harder to deal with. Early childhood professionals can have an important role to play in suggesting strategies for the parents to employ at home with the child. The best results are where the same behavioural management strategies are employed at home and in the early childhood setting. In some cases, the child can be simply distracted so that the outburst lasts only a minute or two. In more severe cases, a behaviour modification regime is used (page 194) where there are clear rules about what is unacceptable behaviour, and these rules are consistently applied. In young children, behaviour modification and time out techniques are utilised. In older children, verbal explanations of rules and expectations are employed as well, with attempts to teach him more appropriate ways of letting off steam and venting anger and frustration.

When to seek medical advice

If the aggressive behaviour persists for more than a few weeks, or seems to be getting worse despite the best efforts of carers or teachers, or if he is becoming a danger to other children, then referral to a paediatrician or mental health professional may be indicated. An early referral and institution of strategies to manage the behaviour in the early stages may prevent it becoming entrenched and much more difficult to successfully manage further down the line.

Prevention

Aggressive behaviour can be prevented, or at least minimised, by good parenting practices which discourage aggression as an outlet for frustration or anger, which encourage respect and tolerance of others, and where these non-violent attitudes are modelled by parents and other family members. In early childhood settings, signs of aggressive behaviour are immediately and firmly dealt with, so the child learns very quickly that this behaviour is not acceptable.

Anxiety

Every child, and indeed every adult, becomes anxious from time to time. This is a normal response to stressful or worrying situations. It is part of the body's normal physiological response to stress or perceived danger. Mostly this state is temporary, and the child quickly regains her normal composure. In a small number of children, the anxiety is persistent and comes to interfere with their day-to-day functioning.

Cause

Persistent anxiety states are usually due to a combination of factors. Children with a particular temperament or personality type tend to be more reactive or 'predisposed' to anxiety. Many anxious children have anxious parents, so there is the powerful effect of social conditioning. If the child sees other family members react in a certain way to various situations, she will likely come to react in the same way. Often there are clear external triggers for the anxiety, which can include real family stresses such as moving house, loss of a job, illness or death, or parents separating. There may be anxiety about separating from the parents. In some children there may be no discernable reasons for their anxiety.

Signs and symptoms

Anxiety can manifest itself in a wide variety of ways. There will sometimes be heightened activity of the autonomic nervous system, with dilated pupils, sweaty palms, dry mouth, and fast pulse. Children may have somatic complaints such as recurrent abdominal pain, headache or nausea. There may be problems in social interactions with other children, or a reluctance to participate in or attempt new activities. Parents may report sleep disorders, or bedwetting, or wanting to sleep with the light on.

Treatment

In situations where the anxiety is in reaction to a known external trigger, often all the child needs is reassurance, and the symptoms recede over time without any intervention. However when anxiety is more persistent, then the issues need to be identified and addressed in a family context. This will often require skilled intervention by a paediatrician or mental health professional. Medications are occasionally prescribed for severe cases, but only by a specialist with close supervision.

When to seek medical advice

If a child is exhibiting persistent signs of anxiety, then a referral for expert assessment and intervention is advised.

Attention deficit hyperactivity disorder (ADHD)

ADHD is a term used to describe a condition which has three principal components — problems with attention, physical overactivity, and impulsivity. ADHD is the most common behavioural disorder of children, with estimates of prevalence ranging as high as 5–7% of all children. It is more common in boys. It has been the topic of considerable media debate in recent years, with some people holding a view that it is not a 'real' condition but only a convenient label applied to children with problems of behaviour which are sometimes ascribed to a lack of discipline and poor parenting practices. There are also concerns about the widespread and increasing use of medications for children with ADHD and other behaviour problems.

One of the reasons why ADHD is a complex and sometimes controversial area is that none of the central components of the condition — inattention, overactivity and impulsivity — is abnormal in and of itself. It is simply the level or degree of these behaviours that is considered abnormal and which leads to a diagnosis of ADHD being made. All of the behaviours that are a feature of ADHD are normally seen in younger children. For example, we would expect most toddlers and preschool children to exhibit a fair degree of physical overactivity and impulsivity, and all will have some problems with paying attention to a task for any length of time. They are considered to be normal behaviours for this age group. For this reason, a diagnosis of ADHD is problematic in children below school age. Furthermore, judging these behaviours to be in excess of what is considered normal is quite subjective.

Cause

It is probable that ADHD is predominantly biological in origin, but that family, environmental, social and other factors are also important. In other words it may be that some children are born with a genetic predisposition to ADHD, but whether or not they actually turn out to have the condition depends on a number of environmental factors.

Many of the signs and symptoms seen in ADHD are also found in children who are deaf, who have an anxiety or other emotional disorder, or who have developmental delay. Many children with ADHD have associated developmental and learning problems, and in some instances it may be that the behaviours attributed to ADHD are secondary to these underlying problems.

Signs and symptoms

The diagnostic criteria for ADHD are listed in the table below.

Criteria for diagnosis of ADHD — adapted from the Diagnostic and Statistical Manual of Mental Disorders (DSM-IV) published by the American Psychiatric Association.

- Fidgets or squirms in seat
- Has difficulty remaining seated when required
- Is easily distracted
- Has difficulty waiting for his turn in group situation
- Blurts out answers to questions before they are completed
- Has difficulty following instructions or completing tasks
- Has difficulty in sustaining attention
- Shifts from one uncompleted activity to another
- Has difficulty playing quietly
- Talks excessively
- Interrupts or intrudes on others
- Does not seem to listen to what is being said to him
- Loses things
- Forgetful in daily activities
- Difficulty organising tasks or activities
- Engages in physically dangerous activities without considering the consequences

The diagnosis of ADHD depends on the child exhibiting a certain number of these behaviours in more than one setting (for example at home *and* at school), with onset before the age of 7 years, and the absence of any other developmental or emotional disorder that might account for the behaviour.

As can be seen, there are no objective criteria for the diagnosis of ADHD, nor is there any definitive test that can reliably make the diagnosis. It relies totally on observations and ratings made by parents and teachers. Some teachers and parents will view these behaviours as simply the natural exuberance of high energy children, while others see them as abnormal and needing treatment.

ADHD leads to social difficulties in many children, with a child's peers intolerant of his impulsivity, inability to wait for a turn in playing, continual high levels of activity, and other behaviours outlined above. At school, these behaviours will interfere with the child's learning, sometimes leading to a cycle of poor academic achievement, social problems, and low self-esteem. In addition, many have associated developmental weaknesses in areas such as short-term memory, fine motor control and handwriting and organisation, which further places them at risk of school problems.

Treatment

Treatment of ADHD first requires a detailed and comprehensive assessment by a skilled professional to exclude other conditions and document the range and severity of the behaviours and any associated problems. Successful treatment is always multi-modal and includes all of the following components.

Parent counselling

Parents are given strategies for how best to manage the child's behaviour, with a particular focus on behaviour modification techniques, where attempts are made to shape his behaviour. Good behaviour is praised and rewarded, and minor irritating behaviour is ignored. Giving clear directions, setting consistent limits, and the maintenance of predictable routines are all emphasised.

Advice to preschools and schools

In structured settings such as preschools and schools, the behaviours are often most troublesome. The strategies outlined above — routines and shaping behaviour — are especially important in these settings.

Medications

Medication is not a cure for ADHD but for many children can significantly reduce the problematic behaviours, and in some instances its effect can be dramatic. Medication may also augment other interventions such as parent counselling and behaviour modification. There are some concerns with prescribing medication to children younger that 5 years of age for the reasons previously outlined. The most commonly used medications are the psychostimulants (methylphenidate or Ritalin, and dexamphetamine). In most states, only specialists such as paediatricians, neurologists and psychiatrists are able to prescribe these medications.

Other treatments

From time to time other treatments are claimed to be effective for the treatment of ADHD and other behavioural or developmental disorders, the most common of which is dietary. For many years claims have been made that ADHD is caused by colourings and flavourings in the diet, both naturally occurring and food additives. It is further claimed that the symptoms of ADHD can be cured or greatly reduced by eliminating certain foods from the child's diet. Although some studies over the years have found some evidence that an elimination diet may help a small number of children, the consensus of most experts in this area is that for the vast majority of children special diets have very little or no place in any treatment regime.

When to seek medical advice

The child's doctor may be helpful in providing advice in the early stages of a child's difficult behaviour, and in excluding some of the other causes that may be responsible.

Prevention

Difficulties with behaviour need to be addressed early in the piece to prevent them from becoming entrenched. Many parents will benefit from advice about the most appropriate strategies to contain difficult behaviours in their young child, and there is some evidence that parenting advice can be very helpful in eliminating or reducing behaviour problems. Professionals working in the early childhood setting can play a very important role in providing advice to parents about strategies to use, modelling for them, or referring them to other professionals for more comprehensive assessment and intervention.

Autism

Autism is a severe developmental disorder of childhood. It is part of a spectrum of disorders referred to as Pervasive Developmental Disorders (PDD), which includes Asperger syndrome (see page 169). It is seen in about one in a thousand children, and is three times more common in boys.

Cause

The cause is not known, and there may be several pathways to this condition. Some recent research suggests there may be a genetic predisposition, and that the condition is due to specific abnormalities of brain functioning. However, at the present time, we do not understand why and how the condition develops.

Signs and symptoms

There are three core features of autism:

1. impairment in social interaction;

2. impairment in communication; and

3. restricted, repetitive and stereotyped patterns of behaviour, activities and interests.

Children with autism have trouble with social interaction. Parents report that from an early age, the child seems not to form emotional contacts with them, or with other family members. They will avoid making eye contact, will not need the hugs and cuddles and physical contact that young children enjoy and crave, and will have little interest in others.

Language is either very poorly developed or non-existent, and other forms of communication are similarly very poor. This further limits social interaction. Sometimes it may be difficult to distinguish autistic children from those who have severe language problems and who become socially withdrawn as a consequence of their difficulty communicating. Autism can also be confused with intellectual disability, which also limits communication and, sometimes, social interaction.

Children with autism exhibit repetitive and persistent behaviours and interests such as hand flapping and fascination with water play and with spinning objects. They will often sit and rock, totally self-absorbed, with very little interest in what is going on around them. Routines are very important to these children, and they may become upset when there is a change.

There is a range of severity of autism, so that the exact features will vary from child to child. However, all will have signs in the three distinct areas outlined above.

Treatment

The treatment of autism is very specialised and often involves the child attending a special intervention centre. Intervention has intensive educational and behavioural components, and parents are taught management techniques for use at home. Occasionally medications are used for specific problems, but no drugs or any other substances have been shown to benefit children with autism, despite claims that are made from time to time.

When to seek medical advice

Parents may be concerned in the infancy or early toddler stage that their child is not socially responsive, does not look to them for comfort, and is not cuddly. Autism is not diagnosed until the toddler period when the other features become apparent. If a young child is displaying any of the behaviours associated with autism, he should be seen by a paediatrician as soon as possible so a definitive diagnosis can be made and early intervention arranged.

Asperger syndrome

Children with Asperger syndrome also have marked communication and social difficulties (see Autism, page 167), but their language abilities are usually intact, and they have normal intelligence. Often these children are difficult to distinguish from normal children who are introverted or 'different'.

Asperger syndrome is the term applied to one end of the spectrum of conditions called pervasive developmental disorders. Autism is at one end of severity, and Asperger syndrome is at the other end — the mildest and highest functioning end.

Cause

Like autism, Asperger syndrome is believed to be due to specific abnormalities of brain functioning, though the exact cause and evolution is unknown. There is a genetic predisposition, and often a family member (usually the father) has similar traits. It is much more common in boys than in girls.

Signs and symptoms

There is a wide range of severity of Asperger syndrome. However, generally these are children who have at least a normal and often a high IQ, and essentially normal language function. There are two major traits in children with Asperger syndrome. The first is their special interest and often obsession in a particular area, such as some aspect of science, history or geography, or more obscure topics such as dinosaurs or constellation of stars. However, the other major trait is their difficulty with socialisation. They usually have normal language skills, but have difficulty picking up social cues or problems taking turns. They may have difficulty with humour, such as laughing inappropriately or not understanding jokes. Often they are frustrated by their difficulty interacting with other children, despite their best efforts.

Children with Asperger syndrome can have attentional problems and are sometimes described as being in a world of their own.

Treatment

There is no specific treatment for children with Asperger syndrome. Intervention needs to be individualised according to the needs of each child. They need support in their attempts at socialisation, and will often benefit from parents and teachers helping to structure their interactions with other children. Frequent and rapid transitions from one activity to another should be avoided as this sometimes causes difficulty for them. Their strengths should be identified and validated, and can form the basis of efforts to maintain self-esteem.

When to seek medical advice

Because there is no uniform presenting feature of Asperger syndrome, it is difficult to be prescriptive about when medical advice should be sought. Parents may notice that their child is 'eccentric' or 'different' in some way, may note difficulty with communication or socialisation, or have concerns about stereotypic and often perseverative behaviour. As in all cases where there is parental concern about development or behaviour, they should be encouraged to seek medical advice earlier rather than later. At best, they can be reassured that everything is normal, and at worst effective interventions can be organised at an early stage.

Biting

Biting is commonly seen in the toddler and sometimes in the preschool period. It is more common in boys than girls, and can be directed against peers, parents or caregivers.

Cause

Biting can be a manifestation of aggressive behaviour, and often occurs in response to anger or frustration or not getting their own way.

Signs and symptoms

It is often early childhood staff who first become concerned about the biting behaviour, as the child mixes with other children of the same age. The child may bite other children, sometimes without any apparent provocation. At other times it might be a sign of anger, for example an altercation over a toy that one child takes away from the other or refuses to share. The child may bite a carer or teacher when he does not get his own way or when he is being physically removed from a situation where he has displayed inappropriate aggressive behaviour. Biting in their young child is one of the most distressing behaviours for parents because of its unacceptable social connotations. At times it is other parents who draw the attention of early childhood professionals to the biting when they hear reports about it or notice tooth marks on their own child which have been inflicted by another.

Treatment

It should be made very clear to the child from the outset that such behaviour is inappropriate and will not be tolerated. When it occurs, the child is immediately told in a very loud voice 'No! You are not to bite!' and removed physically from the situation. He is then taken to a different part of the room for a few minutes. He is then allowed to rejoin the activity with a warning that he must not bite. If it happens again, then the same intervention is implemented immediately. Soon the child will learn that there is zero tolerance of biting, and that there are consequences when it happens.

Prevention

Biting is often seen as part of a pattern of aggressive responses to frustration or disagreements in young children. It is important that the child knows right from the outset that this sort of behaviour will not be tolerated. He should be diverted into more appropriate ways of dealing with frustrations and not getting his own way. Learning adaptive ways in the early years will stand him in good stead for the rest of his life, and parents and early childhood professionals can have a significant impact on helping the child learn appropriate behaviours.

Breath holding

This behaviour can occur in young children from about 6 months of age, and is commonest in the young toddler age group.

Cause

The breath-holding episode is a reaction to anger or frustration, or sometimes to fear or pain. It is not known why some young children react in this way.

Signs and symptoms

The episode begins with crying as the result of frustration or anger or pain. After a period of increasingly intense crying, the child suddenly stops breathing. He may become blue, limp and even seem to lose consciousness. His arms and legs may move as if he is having a convulsion. After a brief amount of time, usually half a minute or less, the child begins breathing again without any apparent after effects. However, it seems an eternity to the parent or caregiver to whom the whole episode is frightening.

Treatment

There is no specific treatment. Sometimes the child can be distracted during the crying phase when he is beginning to wind himself up. Make sure the child is safe and not in a position where he might roll off a bed or fall off a chair and hurt himself. Otherwise there is not much to do except ignore him and wait for it to be over, which is of course not easy to do. These episodes never cause any long-term harm to the child, and as he gets older they will diminish in frequency and then disappear completely.

When to seek medical advice

Some parents and early childhood professionals will have the confidence and experience to take these episodes in their stride, but it is often a good idea to have the child checked out to make sure there are no underlying medical conditions, especially as severe breath-holding episodes are sometimes difficult to differentiate from convulsions. Parents should always be notified if it occurs in an early childhood setting.

Prevention

Little can be done to prevent breath-holding attacks. While theoretically it might be possible to minimise frustration in the young child, in practice this is impossible.

Bullying

Bullying in its various forms has emerged as a major public concern, both in children and adults. It can begin at preschool, though it is most prevalent in school-age children.

Cause

There are a number of children who appear to be insensitive to the feelings of others, though teasing and bullying is also part of the dynamic of group interaction. Often there may be one or two instigators, and others join in because of peer pressure. The victim is often a child who is a little different, either because of stature, physical appearance, temperament or cultural background. The attitude and reactions of teachers and others working in that particular setting is an important influence on the outcome.

Signs and symptoms

Bullying can be verbal or physical. It is sometimes a fine dividing line to differentiate between the normal social groupings that take place amongst children of all ages, where some children are invariably excluded, and teasing or continual and persistent harassment. Children react to bullying in different ways. Some may be aggressive back to their tormentors, but most react in a more passive way, becoming withdrawn and unhappy and often not wanting to go to school.

Treatment

Every setting should have a responsive, proactive policy on bullying, and it should be predicated on zero tolerance. Young children should be made aware that this behaviour will not be tolerated. In developmentally appropriate ways, they are told of the effect it has on other children, and of the consequences if it continues. Parents should also be notified so the message can be reinforced at home. Where bullying has been long standing, especially in older children, the victim may in some instances need professional intervention.

When to seek medical advice

Some children may have somatic complaints such as abdominal pain or headache as a response to the stress of being bullied, and medical consultation will ensure there is no underlying organic condition.

Prevention

All children should be taught the importance of tolerance and inclusion. This can begin at a young age, and early childhood professionals are well positioned to influence them in a positive way.

Cerebral palsy

Cerebral palsy is a disorder of posture and movement caused by damage to the developing brain either before, during or after birth. It is the motor areas of the brain that are most affected, so resulting in disorders of movement, though other areas may also be affected.

Cause

There are a number of causes of cerebral palsy. Problems during birth account for perhaps 10% of all cases, and another 10% are caused by infections in early childhood such as meningitis or encephalitis, or by serious head injuries. Very premature and low birth weight babies are especially at risk. In many children, no cause can be identified.

Signs and symptoms

There are a number of different types of cerebral palsy; it is classified according to the type of motor disorder, the parts of the body affected (whole body, one side or lower limbs), and its severity. There is great variability in how cerebral palsy manifests itself according to the type and severity. Some children are severely disabled while others just appear clumsy and have some subtle difficulties with motor coordination.

The signs and symptoms of cerebral palsy are usually not noticeable at birth. Clues as to the presence of the disorder only appear after some months. There may be problems with sucking or swallowing, or with floppiness or body posture, or delayed milestones.

Many children with cerebral palsy may have one or more associated disorders including visual problems, hearing deficits, epilepsy, intellectual disability, speech and language difficulties, and learning problems.

Children with cerebral palsy cause stress for parents and other family members. In addition to the extra care and attention many of these children need, there are the inevitable and understandable reactions that all parents will experience with having a child with a disability.

Treatment

There is no cure for cerebral palsy. The aim of treatment is to minimise the motor and other problems to allow the child to live as normal a life as possible given her disabilities. Management involves a multi-disciplinary team which may include the family doctor, paediatrician, physiotherapist, orthopaedic surgeon, psychologist, speech pathologist, educational specialist and others, depending on the exact nature of the condition and the nature and extent of any associated problems. Treatment modalities may include physiotherapy, splints, surgery, medications, specific therapies from allied health professionals, and special educational interventions. An individual management plan is formulated for each child and family, taking into account their individual needs.

When to seek medical advice

The child should be seen by a doctor if ever the parent or professional suspects there may be something wrong with her. Early diagnosis and early intervention may result in a better outcome for the child and the family.

Prevention

While we do not know enough about the causes of cerebral palsy to prevent most cases, there are some that we can prevent — by ensuring that mothers are immunised against rubella, that all children are fully immunised against the common and potentially serious infectious diseases, and ensuring there is a focus on child safety to prevent head injuries.

Colic (crying/fussing)

'Colic' is a very common condition in infants and a source of great stress and anxiety for many parents. Research now suggests that 'colic' is in fact not a condition at all. Rather it is a commonly used term that describes the crying and fussing seen in young infants, but which probably has little if anything to do with pain or any gastrointestinal disturbance, as the term colic implies.

Cause

There have been literally dozens of explanations suggested for why some babies cry and fuss. They have included excess gas, gastro-oesophageal reflux, infections, poor feeding techniques, allergy either to milk or to the food a breastfeeding mother is eating, and a host of other causes. None of these is true for the vast majority of babies. In a small number of infants there may be a specific cause found. For example, milk allergy is the cause of crying in some babies, though it is blamed much too often than is really the case. Some babies may cry because of an ear or urinary tract infection, while in others there may be inflammation of the gullet due to the vomiting seen in gastro-oesophageal reflux.

However for most of the infants who have excessive crying and fussing, none of these causes apply. Research now suggests that crying and fussing is a normal part of development, and it represents a transient phase in the maturation of the infant's nervous system. Babies with a particular temperament profile are more likely to cry a lot and be more difficult to console. Parents are never the cause of the crying, as is sometimes implied, but if they become tense and anxious as a result of the crying, this can often accentuate the problem.

Signs and symptoms

The crying and fussing usually begins at about three to four weeks, reaches a peak sometime in the third month, and then slowly improves. The baby is restless, irritable, and does not settle into any sort of routine. He feeds well, but soon after a feed begins to cry and may seem hungry again. He will spend a lot of time just grizzling and fussing, but at times may pull his legs up and cry and scream, seemingly very distressed. Nothing the parents do seems to make any difference. It is invariably distressing also for the parents, who wonder if there is something wrong with the baby and also come often to question their competence as parents.

Treatment

The first thing that parents and carers need to understand is just how common crying is, and that it does not usually represent any specific condition that can be treated. Research has shown that the average baby cries and fusses for almost three out of twenty four hours of the day. Treatment that focuses on medications or changes of milk are therefore usually not appropriate. Because the crying always improves over time, claims are sometimes made that improvement is due to whatever treatment the baby was last given, whereas this is usually not the case.

Management is focused on reassuring and providing support to the parents, while trying a number of physical interventions directed to the infant. An exhausted parent is not likely to be successful in being able to attend to the needs of a demanding, irritable baby. Parents need to make sure they get sufficient rest and regular breaks from looking after the child.

There are a number of strategies that can be tried to reduce the infant's crying. There is no way of knowing which ones are likely to be successful, so it is suggested that parents try all of them sequentially until they find those that are helpful. They include extra carrying of the baby (in a papoose is easier); responding quickly and picking him up when he cries (babies cannot be spoilt); offering feeds more frequently; checking that he does not have a wet or soiled nappy, or that he is not too cold or too hot; offering a dummy or a breast to suck on, even if he is not hungry; singing softly to him, or playing soft music; rocking him gently in a carrier or sling; dimming the lights to reduce the amount of stimulation; trying baby massage which often has the effect of relaxing both the baby and the parent.

Most communities have maternal and child health nurses who are skilled at providing this kind of support and advice, and they provide a valuable resource to early childhood settings and to the parents themselves.

When to seek medical advice

It is always a good idea to have the baby checked medically just to make sure that he does not have a specific medical condition that is causing or contributing to the crying.

Depression

Depression is seen in children of all ages, including infants, toddlers and preschoolers, though it is less common in the younger age groups. It is probably more common in childhood than generally realised.

Cause

It is likely that there is an inherited predisposition to depression, with a number of external triggers which can result in a young child becoming depressed. These can include family situations such as divorce or death, the presence of a chronic medical condition, or difficulty with social relationships.

Signs and symptoms

These vary in severity and according to the age of the child. They can include low mood, the absence of enjoyment of usual activities, loss of appetite, irritability, and difficulty in sleeping and concentrating. Anxiety sometimes accompanies the depression, along with sadness and low self-esteem. They will not be very interested in playing with peers, and rarely smile or laugh. The usual exuberance and high energy levels of children are missing; rather the child is flat and withdrawn.

Treatment

Most children with depression need specialised therapy or counselling from an experienced paediatrician, psychiatrist or psychologist. Some children will improve over time without treatment, especially if their depression is a response to a clearly identifiable external event such as a family separation or bereavement. Medications are increasingly used for the treatment of depression in young children. Careful assessment by a child psychiatrist or paediatrician with a special interest in behavioural and emotional problems is important before medications are prescribed, and close monitoring and regular follow-up is essential.

Developmental delay and intellectual disability

Although there is considerable variation between individual children in terms of developmental attainment, in some children development is abnormally delayed. The delay can be global in nature, meaning that there is delay in all developmental domains (motor, language, cognitive or intellectual, and personal–social), or there can be delay in a single domain. All combinations are possible, depending on the cause.

Cause

There are many causes of developmental delay and intellectual disability. These can include genetic disorders (metabolic diseases, chromosome abnormalities such as Down syndrome or other genetic syndromes). They can be due to intrauterine infections during the pregnancy, while illnesses or trauma during or after birth or in early childhood may cause damage to the developing brain. Developmental delay may be associated with specific conditions such as autism or a number of degenerative disorders. Sometimes intellectual disability is caused by lack of environmental stimulation so that the child does not have the opportunity to learn from his environment. Children of intellectually disabled parents are themselves at risk of developmental delay and intellectual disability. In many instances no cause can be found.

Signs and symptoms

The average IQ of the population is 100, and below 70 is considered as intellectual disability. The severity of the developmental delay can vary from severe to mild, as can the exact developmental profile. The age at which the delay is detected depends on its severity and how much contact the child has with health and educational professionals and with other children.

Children who are intellectually disabled may have normal motor development, but poor language and cognitive abilities. Children with severe developmental delay have delayed developmental milestones; they are late in speech development and not as alert and curious as other children the same age. Parents will often suspect something is wrong at an early age, especially if they have had previous children. Sometimes they will just know something is wrong, even though they may not be able to articulate exactly what this is (see Concerns about development and behaviour, page 201). Severe developmental delay will usually be first suspected by the parents.

At the other end of the spectrum are those who have mild developmental delay and intellectual disability. These children are often not diagnosed until they begin attending child care or a more structured setting such as preschool or kindergarten, or a more formal educational setting such as when they begin school. Their delay is mild and so parents may not suspect anything is wrong, and milestones may be only slightly delayed. It is only when they are seen by an experienced teacher and when they are compared with other children that their delay is suspected.

Some conditions that are associated with developmental delay, such as Down syndrome, have characteristic physical features. Other children may have an unusual appearance that leads a professional to suspect they might have an inherited genetic condition.

The nature, type and severity of the developmental delay will determine the degree of disability the child will have. What is common to all children with developmental delay and intellectual disability is difficulty in learning, both at an informal and formal level.

Treatment

All children with developmental delay will need an individualised intervention and management plan that takes into account the needs of the child and the family. The goal of intervention is to allow the child to maximise his potential and, to the extent possible, allow them to lead a normal a life and support the family. The earlier this intervention begins, the better the outcome. The intervention plan is formulated after a comprehensive assessment in which professionals from a number of disciplines are involved.

Some children are able to attend normal preschool and school, though often requiring additional assistance in the classroom setting. Others will need to attend a specialised setting such as a special school. In the preschool period they often attend a playgroup or early intervention centre, where professionals work closely with parents. All children with developmental delay will need special education intervention, and some will need treatment by other professionals such as speech therapists, physiotherapists, occupational therapists and others depending on the specific nature of their disability.

When to seek medical advice

If developmental delay is suspected, the child should be seen by a doctor as soon as possible. The doctor may order some tests, and will then refer the child to a paediatrician or other specialist for assessment. The earlier developmental delay is diagnosed, the sooner intervention can begin. The earlier intervention can begin the better.

Down syndrome

Because of its distinct physical features, Down syndrome is the most recognisable of the genetic syndromes causing developmental delay and intellectual disability. It is present in about one in 800 live births, and is more common in children born to older mothers.

Cause

Down syndrome is due to an abnormality of the chromosomes, the genetic material of the body, specifically due to an extra chromosome 21. The risk increases with advancing maternal age. The risk of having a child with Down syndrome is less than 1 in 1000 if the mother is in her mid-20s, and rises to 1 in 100 if the mother is in her 40s.

Signs and symptoms

The child with Down syndrome has typical facial features including a flat back of head, large protruding tongue, widely separated, slanted eyes, and a flat nasal bridge. There are abnormalities of their hands, including a curved little finger and characteristic palmar creases. They have an increased risk of congenital heart abnormalities, and are more likely to have ear infections and conductive hearing loss.

Children with Down syndrome are developmentally delayed and have variable intellectual disability.

Treatment

There is no specific treatment for Down syndrome. The needs of the child — medical, educational and social — are addressed to enable them to reach their full potential. Early intervention programs have been demonstrated to improve outcomes for children with Down syndrome, and parent and family education and support are important. There are parent support groups in every state, and many families find these a valuable source of information about what to expect as well as a useful form of support.

When to seek medical advice

Every child with Down syndrome should always be seen by a paediatrician.

Prevention

Antenatal diagnosis is now available for older women. A small amount of fluid is taken from the uterus (a technique called amniocentesis) in the first trimester of pregnancy, and the cells tested. If they indicate a Down syndrome child, the woman is offered a termination.

Fears and phobias

All young children go through stages where they have fears and phobias. These are considered a normal part of development during the toddler and preschool years. Usually they are transient, and may be grounded in reality. For example, a young child who is frightened by dog barking may develop a realistic fear of dogs. Young children will have a multitude of fears — of the dark, of spiders and other insects, of strangers coming to take them away. They may be frightened by something they see on television because they do not have the ability to be able to differentiate fact from fiction.

Mostly these fears are transient, and the child literally grows out of it. However sometimes they persist, although they may not interfere too much with everyday life. Many adults for example have a fear of spiders or snakes, and it does not impinge on their day-to-day lives.

A child's fears must be handled in a sensitive and caring manner and not simply brushed aside, for they are very real for her. Reassurance about her safety is important, and early childhood professionals can work with parents to reduce the fears and at times to desensitise them. For example, fear of the dark can be eased by leaving a night light on, and fear of dogs by gently introducing the child to a docile and friendly dog.

Head banging

Head banging is common in toddlers, with up to one in ten engaging in the behaviour at one time or another. It is more common in boys. Parents and early childhood professionals rate it as one of the more distressing forms of behaviour seen in young children.

Cause

It is not known why some children engage in head banging, nor why it is more common in boys. It may be a response to stress or discomfort, and is considered to be one of the rhythmic repetitive behaviours such as body rocking or thumbsucking.

Signs and symptoms

The young child repeatedly bangs his head against the floor, the mattress or side of the bed, or the wall. It lasts for anywhere from a few minutes to an hour or even longer. While it appears that the child is doing this with so much force that surely he must hurt himself, this is not the case and the child seems to be enjoying it. There will often be a bruise or mark on the child's forehead. However there is never any serious injury or long-term consequences as a result of the head banging.

Treatment

No active intervention is necessary, and the best thing is to ignore it. Some parents and professionals may try to distract the child away from this activity and into doing something else. This is reasonable as long as it does not have the effect of increasing the amount of attention paid to the child and thus inadvertently reinforcing it.

Language delay and speech problems

Many children have problems of speech and language, including language delay, problems pronouncing words clearly, or stuttering. Some are transient, and as the child matures the problem disappears. For others, problems in toddler and preschool children are an early sign of serious, long-lasting problems which will affect the child's learning and communication throughout life.

Cause

There are many causes of speech and language problems in young children. Hearing loss, either sensorineural or conductive, is an important one, and every child with language delay should have a formal hearing test. The child may have language delay as part of a generalised developmental delay, or due to a condition such as cerebral palsy or autism. Sometimes there are neurological or structural reasons for speech and language problems, such as cleft palate.

Articulation problems and dysfluency are often transient in young children, though stuttering is common and is said to occur in about 1% of the population.

Signs and symptoms

The child may be slow in achieving normal language milestones. He may seem to understand what is said to him, but has trouble in making himself understood. He may simply point or make unintelligible noises to make his wants known, or else may make attempts to use language but mispronounces his words so that he is difficult to understand. Many toddlers are dysfluent, and have a number of false starts before the intended words come out. Some children have trouble with speech and with comprehension; these are children in whom autism and intellectual disability need to be excluded. Others have isolated problems with comprehension or with articulation or with word finding. Many combinations are seen.

Most children who have difficulty making themselves understood understandably become frustrated, and behaviour disorders of one kind or another are very common. Some become withdrawn, while many become aggressive. Social relationships are affected as they have problems communicating with their peer group.

Treatment

Children with speech and language problems should be assessed by a speech pathologist. Many will be found to have a transient problem which resolves itself over time without any specific intervention. In some instances, parents will be given advice about how to create a language-enriched environment at home, and the speech pathologist may review the child's progress from time to time. A number of children will benefit from regular speech therapy. The exact type of intervention depends on the nature of the problems and the age of the child. All children will benefit from strategies that parents can employ at home, and that early childhood professionals can use in their respective settings.

Any underlying problems, such as conductive deafness, are treated on their merits.

When to seek medical advice

Any child with a language delay or speech problem should see a skilled professional earlier rather than later. The child's doctor can make sure that there is no underlying hearing problem by examining the child and organising a formal hearing test.

Masturbation

Masturbation is very common in young children, and generally should be regarded as a normal part of development. Self-stimulation begins in infants, who quickly learn the pleasure of touch during nappy changing and bath time. Since touching his genitals produces pleasant sensations, he will do it often when his nappy is off. The young child does not do it for sexual or emotional reasons, but because it feels good. There is no reason to discourage it.

Some adults will try to stop this activity, either out of their own embarrassment or because of perceived community attitudes. In the vast majority of children the best intervention is to ignore it completely. Trying to stop it may only serve to increase the chances of it persisting by reinforcing it. Lessons about privacy and modesty are best undertaken when the child is older.

Shyness

Children differ greatly in their temperament and personality. Some are loud and outgoing and confident, others quieter and more hesitant. Many children hold back, especially in new situations. They don't like surprises. They will stand quietly in the background, often hiding behind or holding onto a parent or other adult they can trust, and very slowly venture into a group situation or new activity.

Shyness can be painful for children, as they become anxious about social situations. For many it just takes time, and slowly they adapt to the situation and then freely take part. For others, time makes no difference and they are just shy and awkward in social and other settings. A child's shyness may be part of her temperament profile, may be influenced by modelling by parents and other family members (shy parents are more likely to have shy children), or may be simply due to a lack of confidence in general or in relation to a particular situation the child finds herself in.

It is best to accept the child for who she is and allow her to move and adapt at her own pace. This can be frustrating for parents who want their children to become independent, and some parents will try to force the child into taking a more confident and assertive position in these situations, or will verbally urge her to take part. This public challenge will almost certainly not help, and may only make her more insecure. Over time many children will become more confident and less shy, but others will retain this trait right through their lives. Very occasionally the shyness appears to be so inhibiting to the child's development and social relationships that professional help may be indicated.

Sleep problems

Sleep problems are amongst the commonest concerns that parents have with their young children. Although many of these concerns have to do with sleeping patterns at night at home, many will carry over into the early childhood setting. It is estimated that up to a quarter of all children will have significant sleep problems at some stage. In many children these are transient, and reflect the developmental stage they are going through, together with the environmental context at the time. In a small proportion the sleep problems persist, and in other children it becomes associated with more generalised problems with behaviour.

Sleep problems at different ages

Infancy

Concerns at this age usually are about the unpredictable nature of sleep, and the lack of a predictable routine. This affects the parents, especially the mother, because of their own interrupted sleep.

Toddlers

This is the commonest time for sleep problems. They may not want to go to bed in the first place, despite parents announcing it is bedtime. They may agree to go bed but then refuse to go to sleep, finding a thousand reasons why they cannot sleep, and usually demanding the attention of their parents. Some wake during the night, and do not go readily back to sleep by themselves. They either call out to their parents, or get out of bed and come into the parents' room. At this age other sleep problems begin to emerge, including nightmares, night terrors, sleepwalking and fears and phobias that may interfere with getting to sleep or with sleep itself.

Preschoolers

Preschoolers experience the same sleep problems as toddlers. Bad habits and behaviours learned as toddlers may continue or become worse. In the early school years, most children will have outgrown the problems seen in younger children, but this is the peak age for nightmares, sleep terrors and sleepwalking. Some children may have trouble getting to sleep, or may wake early in the morning. This is usually related to stresses in their everyday lives.

Management of sleep problems — general principles

Many parents do not understand the normal sleep patterns at different ages. They may have unrealistic expectations of their child's sleep. Children do not sleep deeply all night, but go through a number of distinct phases. During some of these phases they sleep very heavily, and at other times their sleep is light and they are easily awakened. Many children wake during the night, and most will simply roll over and go back to sleep. Many children with sleep problems have never learned to fall asleep by themselves. They have become dependent on a parent being there, or being rocked to sleep, or falling asleep in the arms of a parent. If they wake in the middle of the night they have gotten used to calling out until a parent comes into their room and sits with them until they fall asleep again.

Many ongoing sleep problems are therefore contributed to by inappropriate parental intervention. One of the goals of intervention in children with sleep problems is to teach the child some independence in relation to his sleep. This means pointing out the way in which the parents' well meaning reactions to the child's sleep problems in fact make it worse. This is not to blame them — the parents are not responsible for the child's sleep problems. However, their reactions serve to reinforce and accentuate the very behaviours that they are concerned about.

The child who resists going to bed

Parents need to establish a set routine at bedtime, the culmination of which is that the parents say goodnight to the child and leave the room. This might involve changing into pyjamas, brushing teeth, a bedtime story, and so on. Once the parents leave the room, they do not return. If the child calls out, the parents simply ignore it; they should not respond in any way, resisting the temptation to tell the child to go to sleep. Any response by the parents will serve to reinforce the behaviour. If the child comes out of the room, he is quickly returned to his bed. There may be some crying, which is best ignored. This may be distressing to the parents, but will soon stop. The next morning, if the child has gone to bed with a minimum of fuss, he is praised effusively for being so grown up.

The child who wakes at night

Again the intent is to eliminate the child's dependency on the parents. Two techniques can be used, either 'cold turkey' or 'controlled crying'. Both of these have been shown to be successful. In the cold turkey technique, the child's crying or calling to his parents is simply ignored. Eventually it will stop and the child will fall asleep, and within a few nights the attempts to engage his parents will be reduced and then disappear, as the child learns that his parents will not come into his room. This technique is not acceptable for all parents, as many will find it stressful to ignore the crying of their toddler.

The controlled crying technique may suit some parents better. When the child wakes up and cries or calls out, a parent goes into the room, but does not pick up the child. The parent reassures the child and waits until the crying stops, and then leaves. If the crying resumes, the same strategy is repeated, but this time instead of responding immediately, the parent waits for a minute or two, then goes in and stays with the child until he is calm, and then again leaves the room. This strategy is repeated, and each time the period taken to respond to the child is slowly increased. Eventually he will fall asleep.

The child who gets into the parents' bed

The principles are the same, that is, to teach the child that if he wakes up he needs to stay in his room and go back to sleep. As soon as the child comes into the parents' room, he is immediately returned to his own bed. This may need to be repeated over a few nights before the child gets the message. It should be emphasised that co-sleeping is not harmful per se. In fact it is the norm in many cultures and in many families. There is no evidence that it has any long-term harmful effects on the child. In suggesting strategies for stopping this practice, there is no implication intended that this practice is to be frowned upon. Rather these suggestions are for those families who do see it as a problem and want it to stop.

Nightmares

Nightmares occur during changes in the sleep cycle. They are the same as the bad dreams that adults have. The child may wake frightened and crying. The content may relate to experiences in the child's life, or may be unrelated. No matter how strange the content of the nightmare, it is very real for the child, so reassurance is very important. Usually the child will readily go back to sleep.

Night terrors

These are quite different from nightmares. The child wakes in the middle of the night literally in terror, with dilated pupils and racing pulse. She is usually not aware even of the parents' presence and is impossible to console. After a few minutes the child goes back to sleep, and will have no recollection of the episode the next morning. Night terrors resolve over time and no treatment is necessary.

Sleeptalking and sleepwalking

Many children talk in their sleep, repeating single words, or having imaginary conversations. They continue to sleep soundly. No intervention is warranted.

Sometimes a child sits up in the middle of the night and may unsteadily begin to walk around the house. She is more asleep than awake, with a blank unseeing look on her face and sometimes talking as well. If left alone she will usually return to bed, with no recollection of the event. Parents can gently guide her back to bed. Sleepwalking is harmless, and the only possible harm can come from walking into things. No intervention is needed, and it soon stops.

Implications of sleep problems for early childhood professionals

Some of the problems with sleep may be manifest in the early childhood setting, when the child is expected to have a nap during the day. Some children may be tired as a result of interrupted sleep, with resultant irritable behaviour. Parents may voice concerns to carers or teachers about their child's sleep or behaviour. Where sleep problems are a persistent concern of parents, referral for expert advice is recommended.

Temper tantrums

Temper tantrums are so common as to be considered a normal developmental behaviour. They usually begin in the second year of life as the child goes through the period of establishment of autonomy from his parents, with the inevitable struggle and battles with his parents that this entails. Usually they decrease spontaneously over time and have largely disappeared by 3 or 4 years of age, unless reinforced by parental reaction to them, in which case they may become the child's learned reaction to frustration or to not getting his own way.

Cause

The immediate precipitating event is frustration, either to not getting his own way with the parent or caregiver, or the frustration of not being able to perform some task. Sometimes no apparent cause can be identified.

Signs and symptoms

The child may scream, fall to the floor, wildly flail arms and legs, and sometimes throw objects across the room or kick at toys or furniture. Whatever the exact sequence of behaviours, it is intended to be dramatic, and that is exactly how it is. The tantrum terminates either by the parent distracting the child or picking him up, or if the child loses his audience. The child has the tantrum with the intent of showing his parent that he is displeased. If he sees the parent is not watching or has left the room, the tantrum is usually terminated abruptly. It is only very occasionally that the child is truly distressed.

Treatment

The best way to manage a temper tantrum is to distract the child or to ignore him. This is not always easy to do, for example if the parent and child are in a public place such as a supermarket or visiting friends.
The frequency and duration of temper tantrums are inversely related to how much attention is paid to them. Occasionally the child can become distressed and frightened during a tantrum, probably because he feels out of control. This is best managed by holding the child firmly for a few minutes and speaking softly and reassuringly to him until he is back in control.

Thumb sucking

Thumb sucking and finger sucking are very common in young children. The habit begins in infancy. The baby will initially bring her fingers to her mouth accidentally, and this will over time become more systematic as she derives pleasure and comfort from it. Sucking on a dummy or fingers in infancy is a good self-regulatory strategy, and helps settle and soothe the young child. As the child grows older, she may suck her thumb or fingers in response to stress or anxiety, or when she is tired or goes to sleep. It continues therefore to serve a useful function in the young child.

Some children thus continue a habit that began in infancy; others begin to suck their thumb in the toddler period. Whenever it begins, for most children it is a normal developmental behaviour which sooner or later decreases and then disappears as the child learns different strategies of self-regulation and comfort. There are rarely any long-term consequences of thumb sucking. Sometimes the child's thumb or fingers may develop a callus or even become misshapen, but this soon resolves. In a small number of children where the habit continues, there are concerns that it can interfere with normal teeth development and result in uneven growth. Where this is a concern, consultation with a paediatric dentist is advised.

No specific intervention is needed for thumb sucking. In particular, the use of mittens or hand restraints at night time is ineffective, and appears to be punishing the child for a harmless habit. Bitter tasting substances painted on the child's nails or fingers are not effective and should not be used. If the thumb sucking continues in the school-age child, especially at times other than when she is going to bed, then this may be a sign of an anxiety disorder and may warrant assessment and appropriate management.

Behavioural management, discipline, limit setting

The vast majority of young children will at one stage or another exhibit behaviours that will be of concern to their parents and to the professionals working with them. In fact difficult behaviour is so common in the infant, toddler and preschool group that they are sometimes referred to as 'normal development behaviours', indicating they are part of normal development. Children go through developmental phases where it is known they are more likely to be difficult. For example, many babies go through a period beginning at about four weeks when they cry and fuss a lot, seem irritable and unsettled, and are difficult to console. This is often called 'colic' (see page 176). Similarly, children in the second and third years of life go through a period during which they struggle with the dependency/autonomy balance. They move developmentally from being totally dependent on their parents towards a more independent stance, actively exploring the world around them. This asserting of their independence from their parents has been referred to as 'the terrible twos' because of the difficult behaviours that are almost invariable at this age. Temper tantrums are common and frequent, and child's favourite word seems to be 'No!'.

In the majority of children, these difficult behaviours are transient and self-limited. As the child grows older, the troublesome behaviours diminish (but are often replaced by a different difficult set of behaviours appropriate to that particular developmental phase). Nevertheless, knowing that they are developmentally normal and to be expected, and that they will ease with time, does not necessarily make day-to-day management any easier for parents or professionals.

There are other important issues also regarding behaviour in young children. First is that sometimes parents and caregivers can actually make the behaviour worse and more entrenched. The way they react to the child's behaviour can have the unintended effect of reinforcing the very behaviour they would like to see diminished. This is because the child receives extra attention when he is misbehaving. For example, if a toddler is playing quietly and not causing any trouble, he is usually ignored. No attention is paid to his good behaviour. On the other hand if he begins to act up, for example yelling in a loud voice or swearing or having a tantrum or hitting out at siblings or peers, then this behaviour is noticed and commented on. Even if the attention is negative — the child is told to stop it — it still is attention, and has the effect of reinforcing the behaviour the child was engaging in. The child learns that the way to get attention is to misbehave.

The second issue is the possible long-term consequences of behavioural patterns established in early childhood. Young children benefit greatly from a caretaking environment which is safe and nurturing, where their natural curiosity and capacity for learning is stimulated and reinforced, and where there are clear and explicit rules of appropriate and expected behaviour which are consistently applied. There is research evidence that problematic behaviours that are not dealt with in the early years can become entrenched and lead to maladaptive patterns of behaviour in later childhood, adolescence and adult life. For example, aggression is one of the most stable of behaviours. Aggressive behaviour in the toddler and preschool years, if it is not managed well, has a good chance of persisting during school age and into adolescence and adult life.

The early years are therefore important in terms of having realistic expectations of the normal developmental behaviours at each age group, and understanding how best to manage what are often very difficult behaviours in such a way that they do not become more entrenched. The best results are when parents and professionals work closely together, applying a consistent management plan and set of intervention strategies across all settings. Early childhood professionals can play an important role in helping parents understand what are expected behaviours, and suggesting and modelling management strategies for problematic behaviour that the parents can implement in the home situation.

Discipline

Discipline is sometimes perceived as punishment, but this is not the interpretation that is intended here. Rather the meaning of discipline in this context is teaching young children which behaviours are acceptable and which are not. It means attempting to give them a sense of responsibility for their actions and an understanding that there are consequences of bad behaviour. It means teaching them to be sensitive to other children and respectful of rules. Discipline means trying to teach children, from a young age, that they need to think of the needs of others. Children need to understand that there are limits on what they can do, that sometimes they will not get things their own way, and that compromise is necessary.

Limit setting

All children need to learn about limits. Especially in the toddler and preschool periods, clear and consistently applied limits help the child feel secure as she indulges her natural curiosity and begins to explore the world. As she leaves the safety of the immediate vicinity of her parents and caretakers, she relies on knowing that she will still continue to be safe because her parent or caretaker will make it so. The young child knows that there are limits, even though from time to time she will test them and even protest vigorously when she is prevented from going beyond them. This is part of the consistency and predictability of the caretaking environment which we now understand to be a major contributor to the development of behavioural patterns, both at the present time and into the future.

If there are no limits, or if the limits are not clear, or if they are not applied consistently, then this can be a source of considerable anxiety for a young child. The absence of limits will not help the child to develop self-regulation, which is an important component of good day-to-day functioning. Limits that are applied inconsistently can be bewildering to the child. She does not know from one moment to the next what she can and cannot do. She may become withdrawn, anxious about exploring her environment or engaging her caregivers as she never knows when she is going to be punished, and feels it is better not to take the risk. Alternatively she may begin to act out and constantly test limits, on the basis that at least then she will know what those limits are.

Setting clear, developmentally and age-appropriate limits is therefore a key responsibility for parents and professionals, and something which contributes significantly to the optimal development of the young child.

Physical punishment

Smacking or hitting any child should be avoided. There is rarely, *if ever*, a situation that calls for physical punishment. Apart from the moral argument of infringing the rights of the child, it is ultimately not effective as a way of disciplining her. It is possible, and indeed desirable, to have a well behaved child without resorting to physical punishment, or to the threat of it.

Physical punishment is not as effective as simple behaviour modification strategies in changing or shaping behaviour (see page 199). It may in fact have the opposite effect as it directs attention to the behaviour that the child is being punished for, and may actually reinforce it. Furthermore, it teaches the child that physical punishment or physical aggression is an appropriate way of dealing with others. Finally there is the danger that the person doing the smacking — invariably an adult — is using the smacking as an outlet for his or her anger or frustration. It is difficult to remain calm and in control while engaging in physical punishment of a child.

It is very important to find alternate ways of shaping children's behaviour or of punishing misbehaviour. Physical punishment should never be an option.

Strategies for managing behaviour in young children

▶ Keep a sense of perspective and a sense of humour. While at the time the behaviour may be a source of considerable stress, it is not the end of the world.

▶ Give the child a choice, but set firm limits. The child cannot expect to control all decision-making, but it makes her feel good to be given a limited choice. 'Which dress would you like to wear today — the red one or the blue one?' 'Would you like to have cheese or peanut butter in your sandwich?'

▶ Observe the two fundamental rules of behaviour modification — reinforce wanted behaviour and ignore unwanted behaviour. When the child displays good behaviour this needs to be noticed and paid attention to — it can be a few words of verbal praise, a smile, a tap on the shoulder, a cuddle, or some unexpected pleasant reward such as an ice cream or other special treat. When the behaviour is undesirable or inappropriate, try to ignore it. Any attention paid to behaviour tends to reinforce it. Ignoring is not always easy. At times one cannot ignore unwanted behaviour, for example if the child is being physically aggressive or biting another child, or else putting herself or others in danger. Then the child has to be removed from the situation, for example to time out (see later). However, the same principle applies — pay as little attention as possible to the behaviour so as not to reinforce it.

▶ Plan ahead so the child has some time to adjust mentally to the fact that there will be a change in activity. For example, if the child is preoccupied and playing happily, she should not be suddenly told to stop because it is time to eat or sleep. Rather, tell her a few minutes before that soon she will have to stop what she is doing.

▶ Work with parents to ensure that intervention strategies are consistent. It is confusing for the child to have different rules at home and in the early childhood setting.

▶ Be clear and consistent about limits and expectations, and make sure they are age and developmentally appropriate. There is little point in having rules just for the sake of having them. They should focus on the child's safety and the safety of others, as well as helping the child with self-regulation. There is also little point in having rules if they are not consistently enforced.

▶ Be matter of fact about discipline. Try not to speak to a child in a raised voice. It is more effective to speak to her in a calm, direct way. Stand or sit close to her, make eye contact, and speak to her clearly and simply.

▶ Do not threaten the child with long-term consequences. The younger the child, the more immediate is her time frame.

▶ Use time out when the behaviour cannot be ignored. This removes the child from the action and ensures that she cannot get ongoing attention for the behaviour. The child is warned once and once only that the behaviour is unacceptable, and told if it happens again she will go straight to time out (this can either be in a separate room where she will be alone, or in a different part of the room away from the other children). The point of the exercise is to remove her from the scene and for her to spend a few minutes alone and separate from the other children in the group. If she does not stop the behaviour, or if she does it again, she is taken straight to time out without further warning. The professional talks quietly to the child, making it clear that this behaviour is not acceptable and, where possible and developmentally appropriate, encourages the child to reflect on her actions and consider more appropriate responses. After a few minutes, she is allowed to come back to the group and is treated normally, with no 'post mortems' as to what just happened or why she was sent to time out. Time out is especially effective in dealing with aggressive behaviour such as biting or hitting.

Concerns about development and behaviour

For most health, developmental and behavioural problems in children, the earlier problems are identified and treated the better the outcome. In years gone by there was a tendency to rely on various tests and procedures to try to pick up problems at an early stage. It was thought that if professionals could administer screening tests to all children at regular intervals then this would be the best way of detecting problems. The emphasis was on the results of the tests and procedures that were given to the child by a professional, and the views of the parents and others involved with the child on a day-to-day basis — carers and teachers — was not systematically canvassed.

In recent years there has been an increased appreciation of the importance of parents' observations in being able to accurately identify those children with problems or conditions that impinge on development or behaviour. Research has shown that parent concerns about development, if properly elicited, are just as accurate as any tests in reliably detecting those children with problems. Furthermore it is now appreciated that any parent concern at any time needs to be addressed. While many of these concerns may turn out to be unfounded, or are easily allayed by information or explanation, nevertheless parent concerns need to be taken very seriously. Research has shown that where the parent does hold a concern about the child, there is a strong possibility that she will turn out to have a significant problem. Parents are with the child so much of the time, and are also making comparisons of their child either with older children in the family and how they were progressing at the same age, or with other children. They therefore arrive at the conclusion that their child may be a little slower, or doing things a little differently, and this gives rise to their concerns.

By the same token, any concern held by professionals, or others who are in daily or frequent contact with the child, are also taken very seriously. Early childhood professionals, because they work with young children every day, are in the position where they are readily able to detect development or behaviour which deviates from the normal range. They also often have many years of experience with young children, and a good sense of expectations at each age.

It is important that parents and those working in early childhood settings are able to develop regular and effective communication with each other in relation to each individual child. Observations, milestones, and anecdotes about the child are easily shared on an informal and formal basis. Many early childhood settings set up regular sessions with parents to allow information about the child to be shared more systematically. There is evidence suggesting that where such partnerships are formed and communication is easy and regular, then this provides the best chance of optimal outcome for young children, as well as being an enjoyable experience in itself for both parties. This is a good time to bring up concerns and share observations about the child.

Recently a ten item parent-completed questionnaire has been developed for use by health and other professionals, and has been shown to be as accurate as any of the commonly used developmental screening tests in identifying children more likely to have developmental delay. The PEDS (Parents' Evaluation of Developmental Status) can be used for children from birth through to 8 years of age, and there is an Australian authorised version available (see below). It has been used in Australia by child-care workers and preschool teachers, as well as community nurses, GPs, paediatricians, school teachers and parents. All groups report that they found it useful in structuring an interaction with parents about any concerns they have about their child. While it is designed to be formally scored, with an algorithm recommending what action to take in response to identified parent concerns, it is also a simple and rapid way (it takes parents about two minutes to complete) to elicit parent concerns in a systematic way.

Parents' Evaluation of Developmental Status (PEDS)*

1. Please list any concerns about your child's learning, development and behaviour.

2. Do you have any concerns about how your child talks and makes speech sounds?**

3. Do you have any concerns about how your child understands what you say?

4. Do you have any concerns about how your child uses his or her hands and fingers to do things?

5. Do you have any concerns about how your child uses his or her arms and legs?

6. Do you have any concerns about how your child behaves?

7. Do you have any concerns about how your child gets on with others?

8. Do you have any concerns about how your child is learning to do things for himself/herself?

9. Do you have any concerns about how your child is learning preschool or school skills?

10. Please list any other concerns.

* An Australian authorised version (adapted with permission from Frances Page Glascoe, Ellsworth & Vandermeer Press Ltd) is available from Centre for Community Child Health (03) 9345 6150 or <enquiries.ccch@rch.org.au>.

** For questions 2–9 parents are asked to circle one of three responses — no; yes; a little; and then write any comments they may wish to make.

Family issues
Child abuse/sexual abuse

Child abuse is an area of increasing community concern. It is probable that there has been an increase in rates of child abuse in recent years, though in part this may reflect higher community awareness and higher reporting rates. The incidence is highest in children of preschool age, but it occurs throughout childhood. Child abuse occurs in all social groups, and includes physical abuse, emotional abuse, neglect, and sexual abuse. Anything that threatens the safety and welfare of the child, both physical and psychological, is considered as child abuse.

Cause

The causes of child abuse are complex and varied, but reside usually in the limited capacity of parents and other adults involved in the lives of young children to care adequately for them. They have difficulty coping with the inevitable stresses and frustrations that accompany the task of caring for young children. There are a number of reasons for this. Although it is difficult to generalise, there are themes that are repeated amongst perpetuators of child abuse. Many come from unstable family backgrounds where abuse and violence were present, and often were themselves abused. They have poor impulse control, are quick to anger and have an aggressive nature. Alcohol and drugs often are part of the family culture. Often they have a poor understanding of the needs and capabilities of the child and have unrealistic expectations of the child. The abusing adult can be the male or the female and, in the case of the male, the victim is often not his biological child. There are some conditions which place the child more at risk of being abused — these include prematurity, a chronic medical condition, and physical or cognitive disability.

Signs and symptoms

Physical abuse is easier to detect than emotional abuse or neglect. The child can have a variety of injuries affecting any part of the body. These include bruises, lacerations, cigarette burns, fractures, and damaged internal organs. Often there are characteristic patterns to the injuries that raise suspicion, for example bruising on the buttocks or elsewhere on the child's trunk that look as if they have been caused by a belt or an adult's hand (sometimes it is possible to trace the outline of fingers on the bruise). Often there will be injuries or bruises that cannot be explained by the usual rough and tumble play of childhood, or the parent or caregiver's explanation of how the injury occurred is simply not plausible and does not fit with the nature of the injury. Many serious neurological injuries are caused by an infant or young child being shaken violently, usually because she cries and is difficult to console.

Apart from the physical signs described above, children who are abused may have certain behaviours that may lead one to suspect abuse or neglect. These include withdrawing from social situations, sullen or aggressive behaviour, low self-esteem, and being fearful and vigilant of the surroundings. In addition, they may be dirty and unkempt, or have clothes inappropriate for the weather, or have other features of neglect such as an untreated nappy rash or smelly stained clothes. On the other hand, a well behaved child who is well nourished and looks as if she has been cared for can still be the victim of abuse, and it is important that we avoid stereotyping.

Sexual abuse is when a young child is exposed to any sexual contact or activity. It can occur within or outside the family. It is uncommon for an early childhood professional to observe any physical signs of sexual abuse. Children who are sexually abused will often have some of the behaviours described above. There may also be evidence of developmental regression, so that they revert to behaviours more commonly seen in younger children. For example, if they were toilet-trained they may begin to wet or soil again. There may be evidence of anxiety and insecurity, such as sucking her thumb or being clingy and wanting to be held constantly. She may be sad, and withdraw from social interactions with her peer group. There may be self-destructive behaviour such as pulling out clumps of hair. Finally, suspicion of sexual abuse may be aroused by a young child's language or behaviour being overtly sexual. She may use words describing sexual parts or activities which one would not expect a young child to be aware of, or she may engage in sexually oriented play with other children.

Responsibility of early childhood professionals

Most states in Australia have mandatory reporting legislation. This means that professionals are required by law to report any suspicions of child abuse. Every state has a system covering the reporting of concerns to statutory authorities or to a relevant government department. The anonymity of the person reporting is preserved and as well they are afforded legal protection. It is the responsibility of the early childhood professional to report, not investigate or substantiate, any suspected cases of child abuse. The investigation is the responsibility of the child protection agency.

Treatment

Professionals from several different disciplines can be involved in the assessment and management of child abuse and neglect. The initial contact might be with a GP or paediatrician because of the physical nature of the abuse. The injuries will be carefully documented with detailed clinical descriptions and photographs, and X-rays and blood tests are ordered when indicated. The child occasionally needs admission to hospital if the injuries are severe, or her safety cannot be assured. Management of the family situation is often complex, time consuming and difficult. It involves a careful assessment of the family situation, the identification of stress factors, the planning of specific interventions appropriate to the particular situation and set of circumstances, and plans for ongoing support and follow-up. Sometimes the child is removed from the family, either in the short term or permanently, if it is concluded that it is in her best interests. The safety of the child is always paramount.

When to seek medical advice

A doctor is always involved if there are physical injuries. Apart from initiating any treatment, it is important to carefully document the nature and extent of the injuries, as this may need to be presented as evidence in legal proceedings. Often the GP or paediatrician is a key member of the team that supports the family and the child.

Prevention

Child abuse is a problem for the whole community, as well as individual families. All parents will at some point or another experience exhaustion, frustration, stress and even anger. It is critically important that we advocate for family support systems that help them identify stress points before they reach boiling point, and to help parents learn strategies for dealing with them effectively. Early childhood professionals can play an important role in identifying stresses in families at an early point in time and helping parents understand child development and behaviour so they can have realistic expectations. They can also provide them with practical strategies for managing difficult behaviour.

Divorce/separation

There are an increasing number of young children whose parents separate, and they are invariably affected in one way or another. The way the child reacts to the separation depends on a number of factors.

The most important is the age of the child and her cognitive ability to understand what is happening and why. A young child may have been aware in fairly concrete terms of tension or arguments leading up to the separation, but will not be able to grasp the concept of why her parents are no longer living together. Uppermost in her mind is the fact that she has lost a parent. In addition to the inevitable feelings of grief and loss and sadness, she may also exhibit considerable anger. This will likely be directed mainly at the parent that she remains with, though it may be reflected also in her day-to-day behaviour. She will be angry that her mother or father has sent the other parent away. The young child may blame herself for the separation, thinking that something she did or did not do is the reason why one of her parents is no longer on the scene.

There will often be other changes in her behaviour. She may become clingy and dependent, and will have marked difficulties separating from the parent. Even being dropped off at the early childhood setting, a familiar and comfortable routine, will become a drama with tears and anxiety sometimes bordering on panic. There may be regression in her behaviour. Children who were toilet-trained may begin wetting the bed again, and there may be sleep and other behavioural problems. She may become quiet and withdrawn, or may become aggressive with her parents, siblings and peers. All of these symptoms are a manifestation of the young child's stress and bewilderment. They last for a variable period of time, but will eventually resolve.

Older children have a better capacity to understand the circumstances of the separation and the reasons why. However they will still grieve, be very sad, and have wishes and fantasies that the parents can get back together and for everyone to be happy again. Their school functioning may deteriorate in the short term, as they may have problems with concentration, and some will become depressed. They may become socially withdrawn and have sleep and other behavioural problems.

Generally, the better the parents cope with the traumas of the separation, the better will the children cope. The outcome will be influenced by the quality of the parental and family relationships before and after the separation, and by how smoothly all the logistic and other arrangements can be sorted out. There will have been stresses and traumas for the parents and sometimes for the family leading up to the separation, so the actual event may bring a sense of relief to all concerned, especially if there can be relative harmony afterwards. However, there will still invariably be emotional, financial, logistic and other stresses, and the young child will not be immune from these despite the parents' best efforts. Apart from the disruption to the family routines, she may have to change house, move from her early childhood setting, make new friends, and participate in custody and access arrangements. Sometimes there are major changes in financial circumstances as well, so the child may experience a sense of material deprivation.

The role of early childhood professionals

What young children whose families are breaking up need more than anything else is a sense of security, or predictability, an assurance that they can depend at least on some things still to be the way they used to. When many things around them are uncertain, with many changes, they are anxious there will be more unpleasant surprises. The early childhood setting can provide some of the surety and stability they need at this time. Professionals who have existing relationships with the young child can be a critically important support to her, and also to her parents.

Changes in behaviour along the lines described can also be expected in the early childhood setting, and allowances need to be made for this. The child's parents, caught up in stress and emotional turmoil themselves, will be concerned about how their child is coping and adjusting to the new reality, and frequent communication between the professional and the parents is especially important during this time. It is important to try not to get caught up in disagreements and disputes between the parents, and focus only on the child and what is in her best interests.

Postnatal depression

The birth of a baby signifies drastic changes to the lifestyle of a family. Even in families where there is a division of labour and where there is a great deal of support available to the mother, still most of the burden of taking care of the newborn infant falls on her shoulders. It has been well documented that there often is a drop in mood after the initial euphoria of the birth — 'getting the blues'. This is at least partly attributable to hormonal changes in the days following the birth.

The reality of what it takes to look after a newborn baby only really hits when they go home from hospital. For some families there is a big difference between how they expected things to be and how they really are. If the baby has some difficulty settling into a routine, or if there are problems with feeding or with crying and fussing, this makes matters worse. The mother and her partner may become exhausted and sleep deprived. It is little wonder that some parents have difficulty coping, at least for a while. This is so common as to be considered normal, and usually gets better with time as the baby grows older and the mother and partner get used to things and gain in confidence. This is a time when the family most needs support.

However, for some women this time period is not just a matter of tiredness and difficulty coping; they actually become depressed. Postnatal depression is more common than previously realised, with estimates of up to 1 in 6 mothers suffering from it. It is likely that it is partly caused by hormonal changes, and exacerbated by environmental stresses. While there is a range of severity, the symptoms are similar to depression at other times. They include low energy, fatigue, loss of appetite, anxiety, and difficulty sleeping. The mother's feelings towards her baby may range from anger and ambivalence through to disinterest.

In most cases these symptoms are transient, and last anywhere from weeks to months, and all that is needed in many cases is support and understanding, However, sometimes it is much more serious and psychiatric help is needed. Some mothers and their babies are admitted to mother–baby units of hospitals for assessment and intensive treatment; others benefit from counselling, therapy or sometimes medications.

Implications for early childhood professionals

The infant of a mother with postnatal depression may be attending childcare, or there may be an older child in the early childhood setting. The early childhood professional may see a marked change in the mother following the birth of the new baby, with some of the clinical features outlined above. In these situations the professional can play an important role in offering the mother support and understanding, but also in suggesting she might seek professional help. The community nurse or GP might be a good place to start.

Separation and separation anxiety

Young children go through various stages of dependency on their parents or caregivers. An infant is totally dependent, and the quality of the relationship with her parent or caregiver is a critical one that has an impact beyond those early months. In the first year of life the infant needs the security of someone who is always available to respond to her needs. As she gets older, she begins to venture into the wider world, but always needs to know she can come back to the adult or adults with whom she has formed an attachment. This gives her the security of going confidently out to explore the world and relationships with others. The child's individual temperament plays a part in the way she does this. Some children will be naturally more outgoing than others and will more readily leave the safety and security of their caregiver; others will hold back and take longer to begin to play and interact with other children and with adults.

This understanding of the developmental and emotional needs of infants and young children is why the caretaking environment is considered to be so important in the early years. It is the reason why so much value is placed on high quality child care for infants and young children, with an emphasis on small infant:carer ratios. It is also why continuity of care is so important; the young child needs to form a relationship with one or two carers.

Separation

There are repeated separations that occur between a young child and her parents or caregivers during the first few years of life — babysitters, child care, preschool, leaving her with grandparents or other family members. These separations are an inevitable part of the developmental process for the young child, and allow her in time to develop the independence and self-confidence that will enable her to form relationships with other children and with adults.

Many factors play a part in how easy or difficult separations turn out to be. The age of the child is important, as well as her temperament. At about 7 to 9 months, infants will begin to show separation anxiety from their parents or primary caregiver; this is a normal and predictable emotional milestone for all children. A child who has a temperament that makes her intense or fearful or who adapts slowly to new situations will find separations difficult. On the other hand, some children are more outgoing and relaxed about changes and will take separation in their stride.

Separation of course involves the parents as well as the child. The attitudes of parents and professionals has an effect on separations. Parents bring to the relationship with their children a set of attitudes, anxieties and emotions that are a function of their own life experiences. Some parents find great difficulty coping with crying or signs of distress in their child, and this may impact on the process of separation. Parents may understandably have mixed feelings about leaving their child, especially for the first time, at the early childhood setting. This ambivalence and anxiety can be transmitted to the child, in turn making her anxious.

While separation anxiety will always be present in young children (and in their parents), there are a number of ways that professionals can work with parents to minimise the degree of distress to all concerned.

▶ Encourage the parents to bring the child to the early childhood setting before she actually starts there. Some children may benefit from several visits. The parent can stay there, slowly slipping into the background as the child gets used to the setting, the activities, and the other children and adults who are there.

▶ During these 'orientation' visits, try to have the child meet the one or two caregivers who will be looking after her so she can get to know them and build a trusting relationship with them. At home the parent can talk about them in a positive way — 'guess who we are going to see tomorrow?'.

▶ If the child has a transitional object, such as a favourite teddy or stuffed toy or blanket, encourage her to bring it as this will link her with home and may add to her feelings of security (that is why a transitional object is often called a 'security blanket').

▶ When the parents finally leave her there alone, they should be firm about leaving even if the child protests.

▶ The professional should hold and hug the child and reassure her that her mother (or father) will be back to pick her up, and then after a few minutes distract her into a favourite activity.

▶ Having the child begin gradually often makes it a little easier for all concerned; the child can attend for short periods of time for a few days, gradually extending it as she begins to feel more comfortable.

The majority of young children will come to separate easily after a time, no matter how difficult it has been at the beginning. They will settle into the routines and activities, make friends with other children there, and know that at the end of the day they will be picked up to go home. However, some children continue to have major separation anxieties despite the best efforts of professionals. There may be a number of reasons for this, and sometimes referral for paediatric or professional assessment is indicated.

Symptom checklist

The following is a list of common symptoms seen in young children, together with some of the most common causes. A listing like this is invariably incomplete; it cannot include every possible cause of the symptom in question. It is not intended to turn the early childhood professional into a medical diagnostician; this is the task of the doctor. However, they may find it a useful aid as to the possible causes of many of the common symptoms they may see in young children. They can then check the index of the book and turn to the relevant pages to obtain more details of the signs and symptoms. Again it must be emphasised that this is not a substitute for medical advice and assessment; if in doubt it is always safest to consult with a health professional.

The conditions in bold under each symptom are the most likely or common to be causing the symptom in question. The ones not in bold are possible as a cause but not as likely or common.

ABDOMINAL PAIN

- **Anxiety/stress**
- Appendicitis
- **Constipation**
- Food poisoning
- **Gastroenteritis**
- **Migraine**
- Mumps
- Tonsillitis
- Urinary tract infection
- **Viral infection**

BLISTERS

- **Chickenpox**
- Eczema
- **Impetigo**
- **Hand, foot and mouth disease**

BREATHING DIFFICULTY

- Allergy
- **Asthma**
- **Bronchiolitis**
- Croup
- Inhaled foreign body
- Pneumonia
- Whooping cough

BREATHING NOISILY

- **Asthma**
- **Blocked nose**
- Croup
- Inhaled foreign body

BRUISING

- Child abuse
- Bleeding disorder
- Leukaemia
- **Normal**

CONVULSIONS

- Breath holding
- Epilepsy
- **Febrile convulsion**
- Head injury
- Meningitis

COUGH

- **Asthma**
- Croup
- Inhaled foreign body
- Pneumonia
- **Post virus infection**
- **Virus infection**
- Whooping cough

DIARRHOEA

▶ Food allergy
▶ Food poisoning
▶ **Gastroenteritis**
▶ Giardia infection
▶ Sugar intolerance

EAR PAIN OR DISCHARGE

▶ **Ear infection**
▶ Foreign body
▶ Hay fever
▶ Trauma
▶ Viral infection (common cold)

EYES WATERY, BLOODSHOT OR DISCHARGING

▶ Allergy
▶ **Conjunctivitis**
▶ Foreign body
▶ Hay fever
▶ Measles
▶ **Viral infection (common cold)**

FEVER

▶ Appendicitis
▶ Bronchiolitis
▶ Chickenpox
▶ Croup
▶ **Ear infection**
▶ **Gastroenteritis**
▶ Glandular fever
▶ Hand, foot and mouth disease
▶ Measles
▶ Meningitis
▶ Mumps
▶ Pneumonia
▶ Rubella
▶ **Tonsillitis**
▶ Urinary tract infection
▶ **Viral infection (common cold)**
▶ Whooping cough

GLANDS SWOLLEN

▶ Glandular fever
▶ Impetigo
▶ Mumps
▶ **Tonsillitis**
▶ **Viral infection**

HAIR LOSS

▶ Alopecia areata
▶ **Ringworm**
▶ Self-inflicted

HEADACHE

▶ Anxiety
▶ Depression
▶ Glandular fever
▶ Hay fever
▶ Meningitis
▶ Migraine
▶ Stress
▶ Tonsillitis
▶ **Viral infection**

HEARING LOSS

▶ Congenital
▶ **Ear infection**
▶ **Glue ear**

ITCHING

▶ **Bites — mosquito, bee, wasp**
▶ Chickenpox
▶ **Eczema**
▶ Food allergy
▶ Hives
▶ Impetigo
▶ Scabies

MOUTH SORES (AROUND OR INSIDE)

▶ Hand foot and mouth disease
▶ Impetigo
▶ Viral infection

NAUSEA

▶ Appendicitis
▶ Food poisoning
▶ **Gastroenteritis**
▶ Migraine
▶ **Viral infection**

NOSE BLOCKED OR RUNNING

▶ **Common cold**
▶ Foreign body
▶ **Hay fever**
▶ **Viral infection**

NOSE — BLEEDING

▶ Bleeding disorder
▶ **Common cold**
▶ Foreign body
▶ **Trauma**
▶ **Viral infection**

PALLOR

▶ Anxiety
▶ Fear
▶ **Normal**
▶ **Viral infection**

RASH

▶ **Chickenpox**
▶ **Eczema**
▶ Hand, foot and mouth disease
▶ Hives
▶ Impetigo
▶ Measles
▶ **Nappy rash**
▶ Rubella
▶ **Viral infection**

SLEEP PROBLEMS

▶ Anxiety
▶ **Asthma**

▶ **Behavioural**
▶ Depression
▶ Fears and phobias
▶ **Normal**

SORE THROAT

▶ Allergy
▶ **Common cold**
▶ Croup
▶ **Tonsillitis**
▶ **Viral infection**

SKIN SORES

▶ **Chickenpox**
▶ **Eczema**
▶ Hand, foot and mouth disease
▶ **Impetigo**
▶ Infected cuts

TIREDNESS

▶ Anxiety
▶ **Behavioural**
▶ **Sleep deprivation**
▶ **Viral infection**

VOMITING

▶ Food poisoning
▶ **Gastroenteritis**
▶ Migraine
▶ **Viral infection**
▶ Whooping cough

WHEEZING

▶ **Asthma**
▶ **Bronchiolitis**
▶ Inhaled foreign body
▶ Pneumonia

Index